Basic Maths for Nurses

Includes Dosage Calculations with E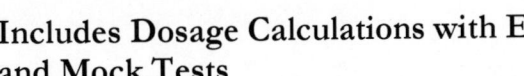 and Mock Tests

By Vali Nasser

Copyright © 2015

E-book editions may also be available for this title. For more information email: valinasser@gmail.com

All rights reserved by the author. No part of this publication can be reproduced, stored in a retrieval system, or transmitted in any form or by any means, electronic, mechanical, photocopying, recording or otherwise, without the prior permission of the publisher and/or author.

ISBN-13: 978-1517357672

ISBN-10: 1517357675

The author will also do his best to review, revise and update this material periodically as necessary. However, neither the author nor the publisher can accept responsibility for loss or damage resulting from the material in this book

Table of Contents

INTRODUCTION 5

CHAPTER 1   ARITHMETIC PART I 7

Addition and Subtraction using Speed Methods 7

Subtraction 8

Speed Method of Subtraction 8

Subtracting from 100, 1000, 10000, 100000 10

Subtracting from 2000, 3000, 4000, 5000, or more thousands 10

IMPORTANT METRIC MEASURES THAT YOU NEED TO BE FAMILIAR WITH 12

PRACTICE QUESTIONS ON CONVERSIONS 17

ANSWERS TO QUESTIONS ON CONVERSIONS: 18

CHAPTER 2   ARITHMETIC PART 2 19

Time Based Questions 19

For converting time from 12 hour clock to 24 hour clock - see examples below 19

More multiplication methods that may be helpful 21

Division 26

DEALING WITH BASIC DOSAGE CALCULATIONS 29

PRACTICE QUESTIONS ON BASIC DOSAGE CALCULATIONS 30

ANSWERS TO PRACTICE QUESTIONS ON BASIC DOSAGE CALCULATIONS ... 31

ROUNDING NUMBERS AND ESTIMATING 33

DOSAGE CALCULATIONS INVOLVING INFUSION RATES 35

EXAMPLES INVOLVING INFUSION TIMES 36

EXAMPLES INVOLVING INFUSION VOLUMES 37

PRACTICE QUESTIONS INVOLVING INFUSION RATES 38

ANSWERS TO PRACTICE QUESTIONS INVOLVING INFUSION RATES 40

EXAMPLES INVOLVING DRUG CONCENTRATION AND PERCENTAGE STRENGTH 43

QUESTIONS INVOLVING WORKING OUT DRUG CONCENTRATIONS 45

ANSWERS TO QUESTIONS INVOLVING WORKING OUT DRUG CONCENTRATIONS 46

EXAMPLES INVOLVING RECONSTITUTION AND DISPLACEMENT 47

CHAPTER 3   ARITHMETIC PART 3 48

EXAMPLES INVOLVING PERCENTAGES AND FRACTIONS 50

PRACTICE QUESTIONS INVOLVING FRACTIONS AND PERCENTAGES............ 53

ANSWERS TO PRACTICE QUESTIONS INVOLVING FRACTIONS AND PERCENTAGES 55

CHAPTER 4   ARITHMETIC PART 4 FRACTIONS 57

Simplifying fractions 57

Finding fraction of an amount 58

Adding and Subtracting Fractions 58

Adding and subtracting mixed numbers............ 60

Multiplying Fractions 61

Division of Fractions............ 61

Multiplying mixed numbers together 62

Dividing mixed numbers together 63

MORE PRACTICE QUESTIONS ON FRACTIONS AND PERCENTAGES: 64

ANSWERS TO PRACTICE QUESTIONS ON FRACTIONS AND PERCENTAGES 65

CHAPTER 5   PROPORTIONS AND RATIOS............ 66

Conversions 67

PRACTICE QUESTIONS ON PROPORTIONS AND RATIOS............ 69

ANSWERS TO PRACTICE QUESTIONS ON PROPORTIONS AND RATIOS............ 70

CHAPTER 6   FORMULAS..71

Formula...71

PRACTICE QUESTIONS ON FORMULAS.. 73

ANSWERS TO PRACTICE QUESTIONS ON FORMULAS... 74

CHAPTER 7:   DATA INTERPRETATION 75

Mean, Median, Mode and Range... 75

Pie Charts 76

Bar charts 78

Line graph.. 80

PRACTICE QUESTIONS ON DATA INTERPRETATION 82

ANSWERS TO PRACTICE QUESTIONS ON DATA INTERPRETATION 84

MOCK TESTS 85

MOCK TEST 1 - 25 MINUTES   NO CALCULATORS ALLOWED 86

ANSWERS TO MOCK TEST 1.. 88

MOCK TEST 2 - 25 MINUTES   NO CALCULATORS ALLOWED 91

ANSWERS FOR MOCK TEST 2... 93

MOCK TEST 3 - 25 MINUTES   NO CALCULATORS ALLOWED 96

ANSWERS TO MOCK TEST 3 98

MOCK TEST 4 - 25 MINUTES   NO CALCULATORS ALLOWED 101

ANSWERS TO MOCK TEST 4 103

SOME USEFUL DEFINITIONS AND REMINDERS... 106

Introduction

This book is aimed at helping Student Nurses to pass their entrance exams as well as Nurses to become familiar with basic maths and dosage calculations with ease. It will also help you to improve your speed in Mental Arithmetic and re-visit some other areas in arithmetic, especially if you did your maths a long time ago or do not feel very confident in this subject.

For nursing entrance exams no calculators are allowed. In real life, although it is sensible to use calculators for complicated calculations, it is important that you can do simple sums with confidence and ease. In addition, I am sure you will want to be reminded how to work out fractions, decimals, percentages, ratios and proportions. Everyday nursing involves being able to **work accurately with dosage calculations** as well as sometimes being able to **estimate values to see if the magnitude of your calculation is roughly right.** You need to be familiar with simple conversions for example from Kilograms to Grams, Grams to Milligrams, Milligrams to Micrograms, Micrograms to Nano-grams, Litres to Milliliters and so on. In addition you need to be able to work out total dosage in tablet or liquid form for a given body weight, interpret how drugs are labelled, and be able to work with formulas given to work out BMI (body mass index), infusion rates, percentage strength, solution strength, and so on. Finally, basic Statistics is useful to make sense of data that is presented visually or numerically in articles and nursing journals. All these topics are included in this book.

I am sure you will agree that it is important to make sure that dosage calculations need to be accurate as the wrong dosage can sometimes be fatal. Hence it is always a good idea to <u>double check your answers</u>. Although a lot of the material in the first two chapters may be familiar to you, hopefully you will find some of the 'Speed Methods' introduced helpful for working out basic questions in arithmetic quickly. This will help you to approach basic arithmetical problems with more confidence.

If you can pass the four Mock Tests at the end of this book it is very likely you will get through the entrance tests required for nursing. If necessary go through these tests several times until you are confident with the method(s) explained in the answers.

One thing to remember is that there is often more than one way of working out a given problem. It does not matter which method you use, so long as you feel comfortable with it.

About the Author

The author of this book has experience in both consultancy work, research and teaching. The author's initial book 'Speed Mathematics Using the Vedic System' has a significant following and has been translated into Japanese and Chinese as well as German. In addition, his book 'Pass the QTS Numeracy Test with ease' is very popular with teacher trainees. Besides being a specialist mathematics teacher the author also has a degree in psychology. This has enabled him to work as an organizational development consultant giving him exposure to psychometric testing particularly applicable to numerical reasoning. He hopes that this book 'Basic Maths for Nurses' will help those aspiring to become nurses to pass their entrance tests as well as help some to refresh their memories.

Chapter 1   Arithmetic part I

Addition and Subtraction using Speed Methods

The normal approach of column addition and subtraction is a good method and if you feel happy with it then you should have no problems with this part of arithmetic. Make sure that when dealing with adding and subtracting decimal numbers, the decimal points are aligned.

Consider the **Speed Method** below for addition

Compensating or adjusting method

In this method we simply adjust by adding or subtracting from the rounded up or rounded down number as shown in the examples below. In example1 we round up 96 to 100 and adjust by taking away 4. Similarly we round up 69 to 70 and adjust by taking away 1. See below for all the working out.

Example1:

96 + 69 =

100 − 4 + 70 − 1 =

170 − 5 = 165

Example2:

59 + 88 + 23 =

60 − 1 + 90 − 2 + 20 + 3

150 + 20 − 3 + 3 = 170

Basic Arithmetic Question

A customer buys three items from a shoe shop, items A, B and C. The selling prices are as follows: A sells for £23.90, B sells for £33.75 and C sells for £19.95. Find the total amount the customer has to pay.

Method:

Total cost = £23.90 + £33.75 + £19.95

= £24 − 10p + £34 − 25p + £20 − 5p = £24 + £34 + £20 − 10p − 25p − 5p

= £78 − 40p = £77.60

Subtraction

You probably remember column subtraction and the number line method from your 'O' level or GCSE days. Before we go on to use the *'Speed Method'* let us revisit the familiar method for subtraction.

Example1:

Work out: 241 - 28

Traditional column method

The traditional methods of subtraction serve us well in mathematics. However, there is one more strategy that we can use to make this process much easier but more of this later. First we will consider the normal approach.

Consider the following example:

$$\begin{array}{r} 2\overset{1}{4}\overset{1}{1} \\ -\overset{1}{2}8 \\ \hline 213 \end{array}$$

Starting from the right hand side we cannot subtract 8 from 1 so we borrow 1 from the tens column to make the units column 11. Subtracting 8 from 11 gives us 3, however since we have taken away 1 from the tens column we are left with 3 in this column. Subtracting 2 from 3 in the tens column gives us 1. Since we have nothing else to take away the final answer is 213.

Speed Method of Subtraction

Example1: Now consider the same problem using a *Speed Method*.

If we add 2 to the top and bottom number we get:

$$\begin{array}{rl} 243 & (241+2) \\ -30 & (28+2) \\ \hline 213 & \end{array}$$

You can see that subtracting 30 from 243 is easier than subtracting 28 from 241!

This strategy relies on the algebraic fact that if you add or subtract the same number from the top and bottom numbers you do not change the answer to the subtraction sum.

So essentially we try and add or subtract a certain number to both the numbers in order to make the sum simpler. A few more examples will help.

Example 2:

$$113$$
$$- 6$$

Add 4 to both numbers (we want to try to make the units column 0 in the bottom row if we can and if it helps) So the new sum is:

$$117$$
$$- 10$$
$$107$$

We can see that if we subtract 10 from 117 we get 107.

Example 3:

$$321$$
$$- 114$$

Let us add 6 to each number so that the unit column in the bottom number becomes a 0 as shown below:

327 (add 6 to 321)

- 120 (add 6 to 114)

207

Subtracting 120 from 327 we get 207 as shown. No borrowing is required.

Note: Sometimes you might find the method above useful; at other times it is easier to revert to the traditional method.

Subtracting from 100, 1000, 10000, 100000

Some people find subtracting from 1000, 10000 or 100000 difficult, so let us consider a useful technique for doing this.

Subtracting from 100, 1000 or 10000 using a *'Speed Method'*

In this case we use the rule **'all from nine and the last from 10'**

Example 1: 100 – 76

We simply take each figure (except the last) in 76 from 9 and the last from 10 as shown below:

```
   1 0 0
 -   7 6
   ─────
     2 4
```

Take 7 from 9 to give 2 and take 6 from 10 to give 4

Example 2: 1000 – 897 = 103

We simply take each figure (except the last) in 897 from 9 and the last from 10 as shown below:

```
   1 0 0 0
 -   8 9 7
   ───────
     1 0 3
```

(Take 8 from 9 to give 1. Take 9 from 9 to give 0 and take 7 from 10 to give 3)

Subtracting from 2000, 3000, 4000, 5000, or more thousands

From the above, use the principle of 'last from 10 and the rest from nine' and 'subtracting 1 from the first digit on the left after all the zeros'

Example 1: Work out 3000 – 347

Using the principle of 'last from 10 the rest from nine' and 'subtracting 1 from the first digit on the left after all the zeros'.

We get the answer to be 2653

Example 2: Work out 7000 – 462

Similarly, the answer in this case is 6538.

Typical Question

At a pharmaceutical company a scientist has 10000 Milliliters of a particular liquid which she uses for her experiments. She uses up 8743 Milliliters after several experimental tests. How much does she have left?

Method: 10 0 0 0

   - 8 7 4 3

     1 2 5 7

(Take 8 from 9 to give 1, 7 from 9 to give 2, 4 from 9 to give 5 and finally 3 from 10 to give 7) This means the scientist has 1257 milliliters of liquid left.

---

i.e take last number from 10
others from 9

all from 9 + last from 10

Important Metric Measures that you need to be familiar with

Volume measures

1 litre(l) = 1000 Millilitres (ml)

1 Litre(l) = 100 Centilitres (cl)

1 Centilitres (cl) = 10ml

Mass (weight) measures

1 Kilogram (kg) =1000 grams (g)

1 Gram (g) = 1000 milligrams (mg)

1 Milligram (mg) = 1000 micrograms (mcg)

1 Microgram (mcg) = 1000 Nano grams (ng)

Notice: To convert **Kg to gm** multiply by 1000, to multiply **g to mg** multiply by 1000 to multiply **mg to mcg** multiply by 1000 and similarly to convert mcg to ng multiply by 1000. Also for **reverse operations** to convert grams to kg divide by 1000, milligrams to grams divide by the 1000, mcg to mg also divide by 1000 and finally to convert ng to mcg divide by a 1000.

Distance measures

1 Kilometre (km) =1000 m

1 Metre (m) = 100 cm

1 Centimetre (cm) =10 Millimetres (mm)

Imperial Measurements that might be useful

1 foot =12 inches

1 yard =3 feet

1 pound = 16 ounces

1 stone = 14 pounds (lb)

1 gallon = 8 pints

1 inch = 2.54 cm (approximately)

Also you are expected to be familiar with multiplying and dividing numbers by 10, 100, 1000 or any other power of 10

Speed Method: Rule for multiplying **whole numbers**:

(1) When multiplying a whole number by 10 add a zero at the end of the number.

(2) When multiplying by 100 add two zeros.

(3) When multiplying by 1000 add three zeros

(4) You simply add the number of zeros reflected in the power of 10.

Some examples will illustrate this:

(1) 45 × 10 = 450 (add 1 zero to 45)
(2) 67 × 100 = 6700 (add 2 zeros to 67)
(3) 65 × 1000 = 65000 (add 3 zeros to 65)
(4) 65788 × 1000000 = 65788000000 (add 6 zeros to 65788)

Speed Method: Rules for numbers with decimals:

When multiplying by 10, 100, 1000 move the decimal place the appropriate number of places to the right.

(1) 67.5 × 10 = 675 (the decimal point is moved 1 place to the right to give us 675.0 which is the same as 675)
(2) 67.5 × 100 = 6750 (this time move the decimal point two places to the right to give 6750.0 which is the same as 6750)
(3) 6.87 × 1000 = 6870 (in this case move the decimal point three places to the right to give the required answer.)

Now consider examples involving division by 10, 100 and 1000 and other powers of ten.

(1) 450 ÷ 10 = 45 (You simply remove one zero from the number)
(2) 5600 ÷ 100 = 56 (This time you remove two zeros from the number)

(3) 45÷100=0.45 (No zeros to remove – so this time move the decimal point two places to the left to give us 0.45)

(4) 345.78÷100 =3.4578 (Again simply move the decimal point 2 places to the left to give the answer)

(5) 456.78÷1000 =0.45678 (Move the decimal point 3 places to the left as shown)

(6) 458 ÷ 0.1 =4580 (remember 0.1 means one–tenth, so dividing a number by 0.1 or one-tenth means the answer becomes 10 times bigger.)

Questions involving powers of 10

(1) Divide 27000 Milliliters by 100   *270*

(2) What is 78.87 multiplied by 1000?   *78870*

(3) What is 67 divided by 100?   *0.67*

(4) What is 687 divided by 0.1? (Tip: Dividing by 0.1 is the same as dividing by one tenth, the answer should thus be 10X bigger))   *6870*

Using the methods shown earlier the answers are:

(1) 270 ml (2) 78870 (3) 0.67 (4) 6870

If you feel comfortable with the methods above you can skip the traditional method below - although if you have time it will add to your conceptual understanding and will help explain why the 'speed method' leads to the correct answers. If you decide to skip the next bit make sure you look at the last part to do with large and small numbers.

Traditional method of multiplying by 10

The traditional method of multiplying by a 10, 100, 1000 is shown below. This method is useful as it cements the conceptual understanding required. Consider having to work out 34 X 10

Consider place value. For example for the number 34, the right hand digit is the units digit and the number 3 on the left hand side is the tens digit or column. In fact every time you move one place to the left you increase the value by 10. So moving left by one place from the tens column we get the 100's column as shown below.

Hundreds	Tens	Units
	3	4

When we multiply by 10 each digit moves one column to the left. So 34 X 10 =340 as shown below. In other words 3 tens becomes 3 hundreds, the 4 units becomes 4 tens as shown. Also notice we have 0 units so we must put a zero in the units column. Moving each digit 1 place to the left has the effect of making it 10 X bigger.

Hundreds	Tens	Units
3	4	0

Consider the sum 34 X 100

Multiplying by 100 is similar. We simply multiply by 10 and then 10 again. This has the effect of moving each digit two places to the left. This makes it 100 X bigger.

The number 34 is shown below as 3 tens and 4 units.

Thousands	Hundreds	Tens	Units
		3	4

We will now do the multiplication and see its effect.

Clearly multiplying 34 by 100 has the effect of moving the 3 in the tens column to the thousands column and the 4 units to the hundreds column. This is shown below.

Thousands	Hundreds	Tens	Units
3	4	0	0

So 34 X 100 = 3400 as shown above.

This technique is important as it illustrates the concept of multiplying by 10 or 100 taking place. The same process applies to multiplying by 1000, 10,000 or a higher power of 10.

Also note, there is a short hand way of writing 100, 1000, 10,000 and larger powers of 10.

$100 = 10^2$ (10 squared, which is 10 × 10)

$1000 = 10^3$ (10 cubed which is 10 × 10 × 10)

$10,000 = 10^4$ ((10 to the power 4, which is 10 × 10 × 10 × 10)

$1000,000 = 10^6$ (10 to the power 6 which is 10 × 10 × 10 × 10 × 10 × 10)

Higher powers can be written similarly.

Small numbers:

One tenth is $\frac{1}{10}$ = 0.1 but can also be written 10^{-1}

One hundredth = $\frac{1}{100}$ = 0.01 which can be written as 10^{-2}

One thousandth = $\frac{1}{1000}$ = 0.001 which can be written as 10^{-3}

One millionth = $\frac{1}{1000000}$ = 0.000001 which can be written as 10^{-6}

Any small number can be written as power of 10 with a negative sign as shown above. Very small numbers are useful in science, for example in particle physics.

Dividing by 10, 100 and 1000

Conceptually, dividing by 10, 100 or 1000 is a similar process, except, on this occasion, you move the digits to the right by the appropriate number of places.

Consider having to divide 34 by 10.

Here 3 tens and 4 units becomes 3 units and 4 tenths as shown.

Hundreds	Tens	Units	Tenths
		3	4

The rationale for this is that we move each digit to the right. So 3 tens becomes 3 units and 4 units becomes 4 tenths as shown above. The answer is written as 3.4. Similarly, when dividing by 100 or a 1000 the number is moved two and three places to the right as appropriate. We will now look at the technique below to work out the answer mechanically. This ensures you get the right answer without having to resort to the thousands, hundreds, tens, units, tenths and hundredths column. The simple rules shown below may help those students who find the above process difficult.

Practice Questions on Conversions

Convert the following as specified.

(1) 6.5 kg to g   6500   × 1,000
(2) 2.5 liters to ml   2500   × 1,000
(3) 6.25 g to mg   6250   × 1000
(4) 0.24 mg to mcg   0240   × 1000
(5) 760 mg to g   760000   ÷ 760 by 1000   0.76
(6) 525 ml to l   ~~525000~~   ÷ 525 by 1000   0.525
(7) 85 mcg to mg   ~~85000~~   ÷ 85 by 1000   0.085
(8) 8550 mcg to mg   8550000   ÷ by 1000   8.55
(9) 660 ml to l   660000   0.66
(10) 3.5 l to ml   3500   × 1000

Answers to Questions on Conversions:

(1) 6500 g (Multiply 6.5 by 1000)

(2) 2500 ml (Multiply 2.5 by 1000)

(3) 6250 mg (Multiply 6.25 by 1000)

(4) 240 mcg (Multiply 0.24 by 1000)

(5) 0.76mg (Divide 760 by 1000)

(6) 0.525ml (Divide 525 by 1000)

(7) 0.085mg (Divide 85 by 1000)

(8) 8.55mg (Divide 8550 by 1000)

(9) 0.66 l (Divide 660 by 1000)

(10) 3500 ml (Multiply 3.5 by 1000)

Chapter 2   Arithmetic Part 2

Time Based Questions

For converting time from 12 hour clock to 24 hour clock - see examples below

12 –Hour Clock	24 –Hour Clock
8.45 am	08:45
11.30 am	11:30
12.20pm	12:20
2.35 pm	14: 35 (after 12pm add the appropriate minutes and hours to 12 hours, in this case 2hrs 35mins +12hrs = 14:35)
8.45 pm	20:45 (8hrs 45mins + 12hrs = 20:45)
11.47pm	23:47 (11hrs 47mins +12hrs = 23:47)

The Convention is that if the time is in 24-hr clock there is no need to put hrs after the time.

Also remember: 2.5 hours = 2 hours 30minutes (0.5 hours = half of 60 minutes)

2.25 hours = Two and a quarter hours = 2hrs 15 minutes

2.4 hours = 2 hours 24 minutes (0.4 hours = 0.4X60 = 24 minutes)

2.1 hours = 2 hours 6 minutes (0.1hours = 0.1 X 60 = 6 minutes)

For other time based questions e.g. years, months, days, hours, minutes or seconds remember the appropriate units.

Example 1: A patient has to take 0.5mg of a certain tablet 5 times a day with an interval of 2.5 hours before the next dose. Assuming the first dose is given at 8.30am. When is the last dose given? Give your answer using the 24 hour clock

Method: Clearly we need to first work out the total time it takes between the first and the last dose. This is 2.5 × 4 = 10 hours. So the last dose is given at 0830 + 10 hours later= 1830. (**Note you multiply by 4 and not 5 as the first dose is given**)

Alternative method: First dose at 0830, second dose at 2.5 hours later = 1100, third dose 2.5 hours later = 1330, fourth dose 2.5 hours later = 1600, and final fifth dose at 2.5 hours later = 1830.

Example 2: In a rehabilitation centre Peter completes a circuit in 2.3 minutes. How many minutes and seconds is this?

Convert 0.3 minutes into seconds. Since one whole minute = 60 seconds, then 0.3 minutes = 0.3X60 = 18 seconds. Hence Peter completes the circuit in 2 minutes and 18 seconds.

(Note that 0.3 X 60 is the same as 3 X 6, hence this is equivalent to 18)

General Multiplication questions

Example1 There are 4 medium size boxes containing 18 black jumpers each and 3 bigger boxes containing 23 black jumpers each. How many black jumpers are there altogether?

Method: 4 boxes of 18 each imply there are 4 X 18 = 72 black jumpers

(Another way of working out 4 X 18 is to break it down as follows: 4 X 18 = 4 X 10 + 4 X8 = 40 + 32 =72)

Similarly, 3 boxes of 23 each means, 3 X 23 =69 black jumpers

Finally, 72 + 69 = 70 +2 + 60 + 9 = 130 + 11 =141

There are a total of 141 black jumpers altogether

Example2

I buy 5 books for £3.97 each. How much change do I get from a £20 note?

Method: Round up each book to £4. Hence the cost of 5 books = £4X5 – 5X3p = £20 - 15p = £19. 85

You can see straight away that I get 15p change from my £20 note

More multiplication methods that may be helpful

The Grid Method of Multiplication

This is a very powerful method for those who find traditional long multiplication methods difficult.

Example1: Multiply 37 × 6

Re-write the number 37 as 30 and 7 and re-write as shown in the grid table.

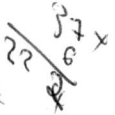

×	30	7
6	180	42

Now simply add up all the numbers inside the grid. So the answer is 180 + 42 =222

Example 2: work out 15×13

To work this out using the grid method, re-write 15 as 10 and 5, and 13 as 10 and 3 as shown on the outside of the grid table.

×	10	5
10	100	50
3	30	15

Multiply out the outside horizontal numbers with the outside vertical numbers to get the numbers inside as shown. Finally, just add up the inside numbers which in this case is 100+50+30+15 =195

Multiplication with decimals

Example3: Work out 1.5 × 1.3

Step1: Leave out the decimal points and just work out the answer to 15×13 as shown above.

We know the answer to this is 195.

Step2: Now count the number of digits there are from the right before the decimal place for each number being multiplied and add them up. That is one for the first number and one for the second number to give a total of 2.

Step3: In the answer 195 count two from the right hand side and insert the decimal point.

So the answer is 1.95

Example 4: Work out 0.15 × 1.3

We know the answer to 15 ×13 is 195

This time the number of digits for each number before the decimal point is 2 for the first number and 1 for the second number giving a total of 3.

We now count 3 places from the right and insert a decimal point.

So the answer is 0.195

If you want to you can think of getting the answer another way:

Consider **Example 3** again: Multiply 1.5×1.3

We know the answer is 195. Note the fact that 1.5 is 15 divided by 10 and 1.3 is 13 divided by 10. So the answer is simply 195 divided by 10 ×10 =100, so we divide 195 by 100 to get the answer as 1.95

More Multiplication

We will look at some fascinating ways of quickly multiplying by 11, 9, and 5, which will help you speed up your number work in mental arithmetic

Multiplying quickly by 11

One common method used is to multiply by 10 and then add the number itself. We will now look at a super- efficient method that is rarely used.

Super-efficient Speed Method:

11 ×11 =121 (the first and last digits remain the same & the middle number is the sum of the first two digits)

The basic method is: Start with the first digit, add the next two, until the last one. This method works with any number of digits.

Let us explore a few more examples with two digit numbers.

13 ×11= 143 (Keep the first and last digit of the number 13 the same, add 1 & 3 to give the middle number 4)

14 × 11= 154

19 × 11= 1(10)9=209 (Notice the middle number is 10, since 1+9=10, so we need to carry 1 to the left hand number.)

A few more examples will show the power of this method.

27 × 11= 297 (the first number=2, the middle number=2+7, the last number =7)

28 × 11=2(10)8= 308 (using similar analysis to 19 × 11 above)

The same principle applies to numbers with more than 2 digits.

Example: Work out 215 × 11

Method: Keep the first and the last digit the same. Starting from the first digit add the subsequent digit to get the next digit, do this again with the second digit until the last digit which stays the same. So, 215 × 11 =2365 (2, is the first digit so stays the same, the sum of 2 and 1 gives you the next digit 3, the sum of 1 and 5 gives you the third digit 6 and finally the last digit 5 stays the same)

> **Example involving multiplying by 11**
>
> In a certain company 54 insurance agents manage to sell 11 health care insurance policies each in a particular month. How many health care insurance policies did these agents sell altogether in that month?
>
> Method: 54 × 11 using the method explained above is 594
>
> Hence, total health care insurance policies sold in this month by these agents = 594 (Method: Keep the first and last digit of the number 54 he same, add 5 & 4 to give the middle number 9)

Multiplying by 5 quickly

Multiply the number by 10 and halve the answer.

Example 1: 5 × 4 = half of 10 × 4 = half of 40 = 20

Example 2: 5 × 16 = half of 10 × 16 = half of 160 =80

Example 3: 5 × 23 = half of 10 × 23 = half of 230 = 115

Multiplying by 9 quickly

Here is an easy method to work out the 9× table

Example 1: Work out 9×7

Method

Step1: Add '0' to the number you are going to multiply by 9, e.g. 7 to get 70

Step2: Now subtract 7 from 70 to get 63 which is the final answer

Example 2: Work out 9 × 35

Method

Step1: Add '0' to the number you are going to multiply by 9, i.e. 35 to get 350

Step2: Now subtract 35 from 350 to get 315 which is the final answer

Example 3: Work out 9 × 78

Method

Step1: Add '0' to the number you are going to multiply by 9, e.g. 78 to get 780

Step2: Now subtract 78 from 780 to get 702 which is the final answer

Multiplying by 12 quickly

Example1: Work out 8 × 12

Method: Multiply 8 by 10 then add to it double of 8

8 × 10 = 80

Double 8 = 16

80 +16 = 96 hence 8 × 12 = 96

Example2: Work out 27 × 12

First work out 27 × 10, which equals 270

Now double 27 (or 2 × 27) = 54

Hence 27 × 12 = 270 + 54 = 324

Example 3: Work out 75 × 12

75 × 12 = 750 + 2×75
 = 750 + 150 = 900

Hence 75 × 12 = 900

The Order of Arithmetical Operations

Remembering the order in which you do arithmetical operations is very important.

The rule taught traditionally is that of **BIDMAS.**

The **BIDMAS** rule is as follows:

  (1) Always work out the **B**racket(s) first
  (2) Then work out the Indices of a number (squares, cubes, square roots and so on)
  (3) Now **M**ultiply and **D**ivide
  (4) Finally do the **A**ddition and **S**ubtraction.

Example 1: 4 + 13(7 – 2) this means add 4 to 13× (7 – 2)

Do the brackets first so 7 – 2 =5, then multiply 5 by 13 to get 65 and finally add 4 to get 69

Example 2: Work out 2 + 8×3

Do the multiplication before the addition

So 8×3 =24 and 2 + 24 = 26

Example 3: work out $3^2 \times 5 - 9$

(3^2 means 3×3 or 3 squared)

Work out the **square of 3 first**, then **multiply by 5** and finally **subtract 9** from the result.

So we have 3×3 = 9, 9×5 = 45 and finally 45 - 9 = 36

Summary:

When working out sums involving mixed operations (e.g. +, - , x and ÷) you need to work out the steps in stages using the BIDMAS rule: So to work out 8 +25 ×12

Do the multiplication first, 25×12 =300, write down 300 then add 8 to get the answer 308.

Division

In general the traditional short division approach is a good method. However, there are some other smart techniques worth considering for special situations.

Dividing a number by 2 is a very useful skill, since if you can divide by 2, you can by halving it again divide by 4 and halving it again divide by 8.

Dividing by 2, 4 and 8

Simply halve the number to divide by 2

(Some find it difficult to halve a number like 13. An alternative strategy is to multiply the number by 5 and divide by 10)

Halving again is the same as dividing by 4

And halving once more is the same as dividing by 8

Example 1: 28 ÷ 2 =14

Example 2: 268÷4 =134÷2 = 67

Example 3: 568÷8=284÷4=142÷2=71

Example 4: 65÷4 =32.5÷2=16.25

Dividing by 5

An easy way to do this is to multiply the number by 2 and divide by 10.

Example 1:   120÷5 = (120 × 2)÷10 =240÷10 =24

Example 2:   127÷5= (127 × 2) ÷10=254÷10=25.4

Similarly to divide by 50 simply multiply by 2 and divide by 100

Dividing by 25

A good way to do this is to multiply by 4 and divide by 100.

Example1: 240 ÷ 25 = (240 × 4) ÷ 100 = 960 ÷ 100 = 9.6

Example2: 700 ÷ 25 = (700 × 4) ÷ 100 = 2800 ÷ 100 = 28

Dividing by other numbers: The conventional short division method is a good method but you might find the speed methods below useful sometimes.

Question involving division

Example1: One particular night a nurse does three hours of overtime work. She gets a total of £67.50. How much does this amount to per hour?

Clearly this is the same as 60 ÷ 3 added to 7.5 ÷ 3

60 ÷ 3 = 20 and 7.5 ÷ 3 = 2.5 which altogether is 22.5

Hence, £67.5 ÷ 3 = £22.50 per hour

Calculators are always there to do complicated divisions like 22.567 ÷ 3.456

However for everyday life it is useful to know how to do simple divisions with speed.

Example 1: Divide 145 by 7

(145 = 140 + 5)

We can say that 140 ÷ 7 = 20, and then we are left with 5/7.

So the answer is 20 and $\frac{5}{7}$ or $20\frac{5}{7}$

Example 2: Divide 103 by 9

(103 = 99 + 4)

= 99 ÷ 9 + 4/9

= $11\frac{4}{9}$

Example 3: Work out 3215 ÷3

3215 = 3000 + 210 + 5

So $\frac{3215}{3} = \frac{3000}{3} + \frac{210}{3} + \frac{5}{3} = 1000 + 70 + 1\frac{2}{3} = 1071\frac{2}{3}$

Dealing with basic dosage Calculations

(1) **Example 1**: A patient needs 750 mg of a certain tablets a day. These particular tablets come in 125 mg stock. (a) How many tablets does this person need to take in a day? (b) The tablets need to be taken after breakfast, lunch and dinner and divided equally. How many tablets are required after each meal?

Method: (a) Total dose required is 750mg. Each tablet is 125 mg. So the total number of tablets required are 750÷125 = 6 tablets. (b) The number of tablets required after each meal is 2.

(2) **Example 2:** This time a patient is prescribed liquid medicine. The patient is prescribed 750 mg of this medicine per day. This particular solution comes in 50 ml for every 250 mg. How many ml of this solution is required in a given day?

Method: Note the units are the same (i.e. 750mg and 250mg). The total requirement is 750 mg. However, 250mg = 50 ml. So 750mg = 250 + 250 +250 = 50ml + 50ml +50ml = 150ml. So this patient needs 150ml of the liquid solution medicine per day.

Another method: Divide 750mg by 250mg to get 3. Then multiply 3 by 50ml to get 150ml

(3) **Example 3:** Anna has been prescribed a certain drug 5mg/kg/day to be taken in three equally divided doses. Anna weighs 63Kg. (a) Calculate her total daily dose (b) Work out her single dose.

Method: (a) Since Anna weighs 64kg her total daily dose is 63×5= 315mg.

(b) Since this divided into 3 doses, her single dose is 315÷3 = 105mg

Practice Questions on basic dosage calculations

(1) Peter is prescribed certain tablets to be taken three times a day (tds). Over 30 days he consumes 90000 mcg. What is his single daily dose in mg?

(2) Clonazepam 0.05 mg/kg/day given is recommended for prophylactic seizures in three equally divided doses. If a child weighs 30kg what is (a) the total dosage per day and (b) what does a single dose amount to?

(3) A patient is prescribed liquid medicine. The prescription is 1000 mg of this liquid medicine per day. This solution comes in 50 ml for every 125 mg. How many ml of this solution is required in a given day?

(4) George has been prescribed a certain drug 5mg/kg/day in to be taken in two equally divided doses. George weighs 72Kg. (a) Calculate his total daily dose (b) Work out his single dose.

(5) A 70 year lady has been advised to take 800 international units of Vitamin D. You are given that 1000 iu (international units) of Vitamin D = 25mg. How many mg of Vitamin D should this lady take?

(6) A patient has been advised to take 75mcg of Levothyroxine per day for his hypothyroidism. (a) How many mcg of Levothyroxine does this patient consume over 30 days? (b) How many mg is this equivalent to over 30 days?

(7) Ahmed has been prescribed 40mg of propranolol to be taken twice a day. The tablets he has been given are 20mg each. How many tablets does Ahmed have to take in total per day?

Answers to Practice Questions on basic dosage calculations

(1) **Answer:** 1 mg

   Method: Since Peter consumes 90000 mcg over 30 days, this means he consumes $\frac{90000}{30} = \frac{9000}{3} = 3000$ mcg per day. This means Peter takes $\frac{3000}{3} = 1000$ mcg per single dose. We know that 1000mcg = 1mg. So his single dose in mg is 1 mg.

(2) **Answer:** (a) 1.5mg/day

   Method: Total daily dose = 0.05 × 30 (dose/kg/day × weight) = 0.5×3 = 1.5mg

   Answer (b) 0.5 mg for a single dose

   Method: Total daily dose÷3 = 1.5÷3 = 0.5 mg

(3) **Answer:** 400ml

   Method: 50ml contains 125mg of the drug. So 1000ml contains $\frac{1000}{125} \times 50 = 8 \times 50 = 400$

   Another method: 50ml contains 125mg. So 100ml contains 250mg. 200ml contains 500mg. Finally 400ml contains 1000mg

(4) **Answer:** (a) 360mg

   Method: Total daily dose = 5×72 = 360mg

   Answer (b) 180 mg

   Method: Since the daily dose = 360 mg, this means each dose is 360÷2 = 180mg

(5) **Answer:** 20mg

   Method: We are given that for Vitamin D 1000 International units = 25mg. This means 100 international units = 2.5mg and so 800 international units = 8×2.5 = 20mg

   Another method: Since 1000 IU = 25mg them 800 IU = $\frac{800}{1000} \times 25 = 0.8 \times 25 = 20$mg

(6) **Answer:** (a) 2250mcg (b) 2.25mg

   Method: (a) Over 30 days the patient consumes 30×75 = 2250mcg

(b) To convert this to mg simply divide 2250 by 1000. 2250÷1000 =2.25mg

(7) **Answer:** 4 tablets per day

Method: Total he takes per day is 40mg × 2 = 80mg. Since each tablet has 20mg, he needs to take a total of 4 tablets a day.

Rounding numbers and estimating

We will start simply with rounding numbers to the nearest 10 and 100

Consider the number 271

Rounded to the nearest 10 this number is 270

Rounded to the nearest 100 this number is 300

(The principle is that if the right hand digit is lower than 5 you drop this number and replace it by 0. Conversely if the number is 5 or more drop that digit and add 1 to the left)

Try a few more:

5382 to the nearest 10 is 5380

5382 to the nearest hundred is 5400

5382 to the nearest 1000 is 5000

This rule can also be applied to decimal numbers:

3.7653 rounded to the nearest thousandth is 3.765

3.7653 rounded to the nearest hundredth is 3.77

3.7653 rounded to the nearest tenth is 3.8

3.7653 rounded to the nearest unit is 4

Tip: remember to use common sense when rounding in real life situations:

Example 1: A hospital ward wants to keep 120 spare empty urine sample bottles in the same size boxes. They can fit 22 bottles in a small box. How many small boxes will they need?

Method: Number of small boxes required will be 120÷22= 5.5 (to one decimal place). But clearly, they cannot have 5.5 boxes. **So they need to have 6 boxes**

Example 2: A patient receives a certain fluid infusion which works out at 30.13 drops per minute. Round this to the nearest drop.

Method: 30.13 to the **nearest whole drop is 30.**

Estimating calculations quickly

Example 1: Work out (2.2 × 7.12)/4.12

We can quickly estimate that this is roughly equal to (2 X 7)/4 =14/4 which is around 3.5 or 4 rounded to the nearest unit. The actual answer is: 3.8 (to 1 decimal place)

Example 2: Work out 38 × 2.9 × 0.53

We can approximate 38 to be 40 to the nearest ten

We can approximate 2.9 o 3 to the nearest unit

We can approximate 0.53 to 0.5 to the nearest tenth

So the magnitude of the answer is 40 × 3 × 0.5

This is 120 × 0.5 =60 (approximately)

Estimating can be very important in case you press the wrong button in a calculator or miscalculate accidentally. By estimating at least you get a rough idea of the answer!

Dosage Calculations involving Infusion Rates

Typically infusion rate calculations involve ml/hour, drops/minute, and infusion volumes.

Example 1: A hospital doctor requests that a patient receives 2 litres of normal Saline over the next 5 hours. What is the infusion rate in ml/hour (millilitres per hour)?

Method: 2 liters = 2000 ml. This means 2000 ml of normal Saline has to be infused over 4 hours. So the infusion rate in ml/hour = 2000÷5 = 400ml/hour

The basic formula to remember in this case is Infusion Rate(ml/hour) = Volume in ml ÷ Time (hours)

Now consider a similar example except this time you want to work out the drops per minute required.

Example 2: A patient is prescribed 0.6 litres of normal Saline over the next two hours. What is the infusion drop rate per minute if the drop rate is 25?

The formula to work out the Infusion Rate in drops per minute is given by:

$$\frac{Volume\ required\ (ml)}{hours} \times \frac{drop\ factor}{60}$$

Method: First note that 0.6 litres = 1000×0.6 ml = 600ml. Since the infusion has to be done in 2 hours this means the infusion rate per hour = 600÷2 = 300.

Finally, the drop factor is given to be 20. Which means the infusion rate = $300 \times \frac{20}{60}$ = $\frac{300}{3}$ = 100 drops per minute.

Example 3: This time a patient is prescribed 0.5 litres of normal Saline over the next two hours. What is the infusion drop rate per minute if the drop rate is 25?

The formula to work out the Infusion Rate in drops per minute is given by:

$$\frac{Volume\ required\ (ml)}{hours} \times \frac{drop\ factor}{60}$$

Method: Using the above formula we can work out the drop rate/min as shown below:

$\frac{500\ (ml)}{2} \times \frac{25}{60} = 250 \times \frac{25}{60} = \frac{6250}{60} = \frac{625}{6} = 104.2$ to 1 decimal place so we round this up to 104. Hence the patient needs to have **104 drops/minute**

Examples involving Infusion Times

The basic formula to remember for working out infusion times is $\frac{Volume\ to\ be\ infused\ (ml)}{Rate\ (ml\ per\ hour)}$ the answer is in hours or of course hours and minutes.

Example 1: A doctor advises a nurse to give a patient 1.2 litre of Saline at a rate of 120 ml/hour. How long will the infusion last for?

Method: Infusion time = $\frac{Volume\ to\ be\ infused\ (ml)}{Rate\ (ml\ per\ hour)}$ = $\frac{1200\ (ml)}{120\ (ml\ per\ hour)}$ = 10 hours

Example 2: A particular patent receives 150ml of fluid at a rate of 300ml.hour. How long will the infusion last for in minutes?

Method: Infusion time = $\frac{Volume\ to\ be\ infused\ (ml)}{Rate\ (ml\ per\ hour)}$ = $\frac{150\ (ml)}{300\ (ml\ per\ hour)}$ = 0.5 hours
= $\frac{1}{2}$ hour = 30 minutes.

Examples involving Infusion Volumes

The formula for calculating infusion volumes is: Volume = Rate (ml/hour) × total running time (hours). The answer can be in ml or litres as appropriate.

Example 1: George is given Saline for a total of 12 hours at the rate of 125ml/hour. How many litres of Saline does George receive?

Method: Volume = Rate (ml/hour) × total running time (hours)

So George receives **125×12 ml = 1500 ml = 1.5 litres**

Example 2: Jessica is given a particular solution at the rate of 250 ml/hour. The infusion lasts for 5 hours. How much of the solution will be infused?

Jessica will receive a total of **250×5 ml = 1250ml or 1.25 litres.**

Example 3: Mohammed receives 100 ml/hr of a particular fluid for 8.5 hours. How many litres of this fluid will be infused in this time period?

Mohammed receives a total of **100×8.5 ml = 850 ml**

Practice Questions involving infusion rates

Questions involving infusion Rates in (ml/hour) $= \dfrac{Volume\ required\ (ml)}{Time\ (hours)}$

(1) 600 ml of fluid is to be infused over 3 hours? Calculate the infusion rate in ml/hour.

(2) A patient receives 1.2 liters of dextrose over 4 hours. What is the infusion rate in ml/hour?

(3) What is the rate in ml/hour if 15ml of fluid is given over 20 minutes?

(4) A patient in a particular ward receives 0.06 liters of Saline which is to be infused over 30 minutes. What is the rate in ml/hour?

Questions involving finding drop rates per minute. Use the formula:

Infusion Rate in drops per minute $= \dfrac{Volume\ required\ (ml)}{hours} \times \dfrac{drop\ factor}{60}$

(5) 1.2 liters of fluid is to be given over 6 hours. What is the infusion rate in drops per minute if the drop factor is 15?

(6) Claire is given 720 ml of dextrose 5% over 6 hours. Calculate the infusion rate in drops per minute if the drop factor is 30.

(7) A child is to receive 1.2 liters of fluid over 10 hours. What is the infusion rate in drops/minute if the drop factor is 20?

(8) 150 ml of blood is to be infused over 2 hours. What is the infusion rate in drops/minute if the drop factor is 20

Questions involving Infusion Times

The basic formula to remember for working out infusion times is

$$\frac{Volume\ to\ be\ infused\ (ml)}{Rate\ (ml\ per\ hour)}$$

(9) A patient is given 600 ml of a solution at the rate of 200ml/hour. How long will the infusion last?

(10) 0.5 liters of Saline is given at the rate of 250ml/hour. How long will the infusion last for?

(11) 1.5 liters of a particular fluid is given at an infusion rate of 200 ml/hour. How long will the infusion last in hours and minutes?

(12) An infusion of 1 liter of Saline starts at 11am. The infusion rate is 250ml/hour. When does the infusion of Saline finish. Give your answer using the 24 hour clock.

Questions involving working out Infusion Volumes:

The formula for working out infusion volume is given by: Volume = Rate (ml/hour) × total running time (hours). The answer can be in ml or litres as appropriate

(13) A certain fluid is given at the rate of 100ml/hour for 45 minutes. How many ml of fluid does this patient receive?

(14) Dextrose 5% is infused at a rate of 80ml/hour. How much dextrose is infused after 10 hours and 30 minutes?

(15) Mary needs blood infusion which is given at a rate of 150ml/hour for 8 hours. How much blood does Mary receive? Give your answer in liters.

(16) A patient is given Saline for 12 hours and 30 minutes at the rate of 125ml.hour. How many liters of Saline does the patient receive altogether in liters? Give your answer to two decimal places

Answers to Practice Questions involving infusion rates

Questions involving infusion Rates in (ml/hour) $= \dfrac{Volume\ required\ (ml)}{Time\ (hours)}$

(1) 600 ml of fluid is to be infused over 3 hours? Calculate the infusion rate in ml/hour.

Answer: 200ml/hour

Method: Using the formula: $\dfrac{Volume\ required\ (ml)}{Time\ (hours)} = \dfrac{600\ (ml)}{3\ (hours)} = 200\text{ml/hr}$

(2) **Answer:** 300ml/hour

Method: Using the formula: $\dfrac{Volume\ required\ (ml)}{Time\ (hours)} = \dfrac{1200\ (ml)}{4\ (hours)} = 300\text{ml/hr}$

(3) **Answer:** 45 ml/hour

Method: Using the formula: $\dfrac{Volume\ required\ (ml)}{Time\ (hours)} = 15 \div \dfrac{1}{3} = 15 \times 3 = 45 \text{ ml/hr}$

Note: 20 minutes $= \dfrac{20}{60} = \dfrac{2}{6} = \dfrac{1}{3}$ hours

(4) **Answer:** 120ml/hour

Method: Using the formula: $\dfrac{Volume\ required\ (ml)}{Time\ (hours)} = \dfrac{60\ ml}{0.5\ hours} = 120 \text{ ml/hour}$

Answers to Questions involving finding drop rates per minute. Use the formula:

Infusion Rate in drops per minute $= \dfrac{Volume\ required\ (ml)}{hours} \times \dfrac{drop\ factor}{60}$

(5) **Answer:** 50 drops/minute

Method: Using the formula to work out drops/min

$\dfrac{Volume\ required\ (ml)}{hours} \times \dfrac{drop\ factor}{60} = \dfrac{1200\ (ml)}{6} \times \dfrac{15}{60} = 200 \times \dfrac{1}{4} = 50 \text{ drops/min}$

(6) **Answer:** 60 drops/minute

Method: Using the formula to work out drops/min

$$\frac{Volume\ required\ (ml)}{hours} \times \frac{drop\ factor}{60} = \frac{720\ (ml)}{6} \times \frac{30}{60} = 120 \times \frac{1}{2} = 60 \text{ drops/min}$$

(7) Answer: 40 drops/minute

Method: Using the formula to work out drops/min

$$\frac{Volume\ required\ (ml)}{hours} \times \frac{drop\ factor}{60} = \frac{1200\ (ml)}{10} \times \frac{20}{60} = 120 \times \frac{1}{3} = 40 \text{ drops/min}$$

(8) Answer: 26 drops/minute

Method: Using the formula to work out drops/min

$$\frac{Volume\ required\ (ml)}{hours} \times \frac{drop\ factor}{60} = \frac{150\ (ml)}{2} \times \frac{20}{60} = 75 \times \frac{1}{3} = 25 \text{ drops/min}$$

Answers to Questions involving Infusion Times

The basic formula to remember for working out infusion times is $\frac{Volume\ to\ be\ infused\ (ml)}{Rate\ (ml\ per\ hour)}$

(9) Answer: 3 hours

Method: Using the formula $\frac{Volume\ to\ be\ infused\ (ml)}{Rate\ (ml\ per\ hour)} = \frac{600\ (ml)}{200\ (ml\ per\ hour)} = 3$ hours

(10) Answer: 2 hours

Method: Using the formula $\frac{Volume\ to\ be\ infused\ (ml)}{Rate\ (ml\ per\ hour)} = \frac{500\ (ml)}{250\ (ml\ per\ hour)} =$ 2hrs

(11) Answer: 7 hours 30 minutes or 7.5 hours

Method: Using the formula $\frac{Volume\ to\ be\ infused\ (ml)}{Rate\ (ml\ per\ hour)} = \frac{1500\ (ml)}{200\ (ml\ per\ hour)} =$ 7.5 hours

(12) **Answer:** 1500 (Using the 24 hour clock)

Method: Using the formula $\frac{Volume\ to\ be\ infused\ (ml)}{Rate\ (ml\ per\ hour)} = \frac{1000\ (ml)}{250\ (ml\ per\ hour)} = 4$ hours. Start time is 11am so end time is 1500.

Answers to Questions involving Infusion Volumes:

The formula to working out infusion volume is given by: Volume = Rate (ml/hour) × total running time (hours). The answer can be in ml or litres as appropriate

(13) **Answer:** 75ml

Method: Volume = Rate (ml/hour) × total running time (hours), so Volume = $100 \times \frac{3}{4}$ (Since 45 minutes is $\frac{3}{4}$ of an hour). $100 \times \frac{3}{4} = 75$ml

(14) **Answer:** 840ml

Method: Volume = Rate (ml/hour) × total running time (hours), so Volume = 80×10.5 (Since 10hours 30 minutes = 10.5 hours). 80×10.5 = 800 + 40 = 840ml

(15) **Answer:** 1.2 litres

Method: Volume = Rate (ml/hour) × total running time (hours), so Volume = 150×8 = 1200 ml = 1200÷1000 litres = 1.2 litres

(16) **Answer:** 15.63 litres

Method: Volume = Rate (ml/hour) × total running time (hours), so Volume = 125×12.5 (Since 12 hours 30minutes is 12.5 hours). 125×12.5 = 15625ml = 15.625 litres = 15.63 litres (to 2 decimal places)

Examples involving drug concentration and percentage strength

Concentration is how strong a solution is. It says whether a certain quantity of solution has more or less of the drug. For example two table spoons of sugar in a glass of water has more sugar than one table spoon of sugar in a glass with the same amount of water In other words the former has a higher concentration of sugar than the latter. Some examples below will illustrate this concept in reality.

Example 1: The concentration of a drug is 0.2 mg/ml. How many mg of the drug are there in 0.5 litres?

Method: 0.5 litres = 1000×0.5 = 500 ml. So the concentration of the drug in 0.5 litres is 500×0.2 = 100mg

Example 2: Another drug has a concentration of 500mg/ml. How many **grams** are there in 200ml of this solution?

Method: 500mg/ml = 0.5g/ml (500 ÷1000). So 200ml has 200×0.5 = **100 grams** of this drug

Above we did some examples on simple drug concentration. Now let us look at some other examples on concentration strength or <u>percentage strength of infusion fluids</u>, recap that solutions stored in <u>concentrated form are known as stock</u>. These solutions can then be diluted to a given strength also expressed in <u>percentage strength in g/100ml or appropriate units</u>.

Example 3: A patient receives 1 litre of 5% dextrose solution. How many grams of dextrose will the patient receive?

Method: In this case we need to work out volume strength ×percentage strength

$= 1000 \times \frac{5}{100} = 50$mg of dextrose

Example 4: 0.5 litres of Saline solution (or more technically a solution that has Sodium Chloride) has a concentration of 0.4% w/v **(w/v means % weight per volume)**. How many grams of Sodium Chloride are there in this 0.5 litres of Saline solution?

Method: 0.4% means 4g/100ml. (remember the concentration in this case is expressed in w/v). This means 500 ml has $500 \times \frac{4}{100}$ = **20 g of Sodium Chloride**

Example 5: A certain solution contains a drug which has a strength of 0.2% w/v. How many mg of this drug are there in 20ml of this solution?

Method: 0.2% means 0.2g/100ml. Now we know that 0.2g = 0.2×1000 = 200mg. This means if 100ml has 200mg, then 20ml has $\frac{20}{100} = \frac{1}{5}$ of 200mg = 40mg of this drug.

N.B. To clarify V/V and W/V a bit more consider the examples below

V/V means volume/volume – see example below

(1) If you have 10% V/V solution of a drug and the patient requires 20ml of the drug. How much of the solution is required?

Method: 10% V/V means for every 100 ml of this solution we have 10 ml of this drug. So if the patient requires 20ml we need $\frac{20}{10} \times 100 = 200$ ml of this solution

W/V means weight/volume – see example below

(2) A certain drug comes in a W/V solution of 6%. The patient requires 18 grams of this drug. How many ml of this solution is required?

Method: 6% W/V means for every 100ml of this solution there 6 grams of this drug. Since the patient requires 18gms, this = $\frac{18}{6} \times 100 = 3 \times 100 = 300$ml

Questions involving working out drug concentrations

(1) A certain concentration of 25 ml contains 50mg of a particular drug. What is the concentration in mg/ml?

(2) A patient receives 1.5 litres of 2% dextrose solution. How many grams of dextrose will the patient receive?

(3) A certain solution contains a drug which has a strength of 0.5% w/v. How many mg of this drug are there in 300ml of this solution?

(4) A solution contains a drug which has a strength of 0.3% w/v. How many mg of this drug are there in 40ml of this solution?

(5) 0.6 litres of a solution of Sodium Chloride has a concentration of 0.4% w/v (w/v means weight per volume). How many g of Sodium Chloride are there in this 0.6 litres of Saline solution?

Answers to Questions involving working out drug concentrations

(1) **Answer**: 2mg/ml

Method: Since 25 ml contains 50mg, it means 1ml would need 50÷25 = 2mg/ml

(2) **Answer**: 30g

Method: In this case we need to work out volume strength ×percentage strength. Remember 2% strength means 2g/100ml. So in this case we work out: $1500 \times \frac{2}{100}$ = 30g of dextrose

(3) **Answer**: 1.5g

Method: 0.5% means 0.5g/100ml. (the concentration in this case is expressed in w/v). This means 300 ml has $300 \times \frac{0.5}{100}$ = 1.5g of this drug

(4) **Answer**: 120mg

Method: 0.3% means 0.3g/100ml. Now we know that 0.3g =0.3×1000 = 300mg. This means if 100 ml has 300mg, so 40ml has $\frac{40}{100} \times 300mg$ = 120mg of this drug.

(5) **Answer**: 2.4 g

Method: 0.4% means 0.4g/100ml. (the concentration in this case is expressed in w/v).But 0.4g = 400mg. This means 600 ml has $\frac{600}{100} \times 400mg$ = 2400 mg of Sodium Chloride = 2.4 g.

Examples involving reconstitution and displacement

Reconstitution: This is simply the process of mixing or diluting solutions. For example when a medication is supplied in powder form it usually has to be mixed with a liquid before administration.

Displacement: This is the increase in volume caused by the displacement value of the powder.

Example 1: 100 mg of a drug in powder is reconstituted with 4.5 ml of sterile water for an injection. The displacement volume is 0.5ml. What volume needs to be administered for a dose of 60mg?

Method: Total volume of the solution including amount displaced = 4.5 + 0.5 = 5ml. Since 5ml now consists of 100mg this means the volume required to administer 60mg is: $\frac{60}{100} \times 5 = 0.6 \times 5 =$ **3ml**

Example 2: One 800mg vial of a certain powder is mixed with 5.3ml of sterile water for an injection. If the displacement volume is 0.7ml what volume is required for a dose of 200mg?

Method: Total volume of the solution including amount displaced = 5.3 + 0.7 = 6ml. Since 6ml is now equivalent to a dose of 800mg. This means the volume required for 600mg is $\frac{200}{800} \times 6 = \frac{2}{8} \times 6 = \frac{1}{4} \times 6 =$ **1.5ml**

Chapter 3   Arithmetic Part 3

Fractions, decimals and percentages

I am sure most of you are aware that $\frac{1}{2}$ = 0.5. This in turn is equal to 50%.

It is worth reviewing this fact. In addition, you should try and remember the following other equivalences if you have forgotten them.

Fractions, decimals and percentage equivalents

Fractions	Decimal	Percentage
$\frac{1}{2}$	0.5	50%
$\frac{1}{4}$	0.25	25%
$\frac{3}{4}$	0.75	75%
$\frac{1}{10}$	0.1	10%
$\frac{1}{5}$	0.2	20%

If we know $\frac{1}{2}$ = 0.5

We can deduce that $\frac{1}{4}$ = 0.25

(Since a quarter is half of half)

Similarly $\frac{1}{8}$ is **0.125**

We can do this quickly because all we do is halve each decimal value.

Half of 0.5 is 0.25, Half of 0.25 is 0.125

We can of course continue this process.

Further if we know $\frac{1}{10}$ **=0.1 we can now work out** $\frac{2}{10}, \frac{3}{10}, \frac{7}{10}$ **etc.**

$\frac{2}{10}$ = 0.2 (2 × 0.1), $\frac{3}{10}$ = 0.3 (3 × 0.1, $\frac{7}{10}$ = 0.7 (7 × 0.1), $\frac{9}{10}$ = 0.9 (9 × 0.1)

Another useful fraction and decimal equivalent to remember is $\frac{1}{3}$=0.333... (0.3 recurring)

The key equivalent percentages to remember are as follows:

$\frac{3}{4}$ = 75%, $\frac{1}{2}$ =50%, $\frac{1}{4}$ = 25%, $\frac{1}{8}$ = 12.5%, $\frac{1}{10}$ = 10%

See summary box below

Summary:

Remember the following equivalences

$\frac{1}{2}$=0.5=50%, $\frac{1}{4}$=0.25=25%, $\frac{3}{4}$=0.75=75%, $\frac{1}{10}$=0.1=10%

Also if you can try to remember, $\frac{1}{5}$=0.2 = 20%, and $\frac{2}{5}$=0.4 =40%, $\frac{1}{3}$=0.333... (0.3 recurring) = 33.33% (to 2 decimal places)

To convert a fraction into a percentage, simply multiply the fraction by 100

Examples involving percentages and fractions

Example 1: Find 25% of £250

Method: Find 50% of £250 and halve it again.

Half of £250 = £125, Half of £125 =£62.50, so 25% of £250 = £62.50

Example 2: In a survey of 50 people the number of people over 60 years of age who took Statins was found to be 19 people.

(1) What fraction of this particular sample took Statins?

(2) What percentage is this?

(1) The survey was done on 50 people. Since 19 people took Statins, the **corresponding fraction is** $\frac{19}{50}$

(2) The percentage of people in this sample that took Statins is $\frac{19}{50} \times 100$ = **38%**, (Divide 100 by 50 to get 2. Then multiply 19 by 2 to get 38%)

Example 3: A patient on 10mg of diazepam per day is asked to gradually reduce his intake. In the first week he is asked to reduce his intake by 20%. How many mg of diazepam does the patient need to take in the first week?

Method: 20% of 10mg is 2mg. ($\frac{20}{100} \times 10 = \frac{200}{100} = 2$). So the **reduction in dosage is 2mg** which means the patient has to take **8mg of diazepam** for the first week as part of his reduction strategy.

Working out increase or decrease in percentages from original value

Example1: In a certain corner shop 16 packs of cereal A were sold in week 1. In the same shop 20 packs of the same cereal were sold in week 2. What was the percentage increase in the cereal packs A sold from week 1 to week 2?

Method: Increase in number of cereal packs A = 20 – 16 = 4. Original number of cereal packs = 16. The increase of 4 was based on 16 cereal packs. To work out the percentage increase we simply divide the increase by the original number of cereal packs and multiply this by 100. That is $\frac{4}{16} \times 100 = \frac{1}{4} \times 100 = 25\%$

To work out decrease in percentages (uses the same principle as above)

Example2: The original price of a projector was: £150, the new price is reduced to £135. What is the percentage decrease in price? The decrease in price is £150 - £135 = £15. The decrease over the original price is $\frac{15}{150}$. To turn this into a percentage we multiply $\frac{15}{150} \times 100 = \frac{1500}{150} = 10\%$. So the decrease in percentage price is 10%.

The basic formula to work out increase or decrease percentage change is shown below:

$$\frac{difference\ between\ final\ and\ original\ value}{original\ value} \times 100$$

One thing to remember though is that the **increase or decrease in percentage points** is different from **increase or decrease in percentages**.

To illustrate this consider the example below:

The unemployment rate in a region A was 8% in 2010. In 2011 the unemployment rate in the same region was 10%. **(1)** What was the **percentage point** increase in unemployment from 2010 to 2011? **(2)** What is the **percentage increase** in unemployment from 2010 to 2011?

(1) The **percentage point** increase is simply 2% (i.e. from 8% to 10%)

(2) However the **percentage increase** in unemployment is $\frac{2}{8} \times 100 = \frac{200}{8} = \frac{100}{4} = 25\%$.

If you are asked to work out the **percentage point increase,** say in sales in Product A changing from 20% to 30%. The answer is obviously 10%. But if asked to work out the **percentage increase**, then the answer is $\frac{10}{20} \times 00 = \frac{1000}{20} = \frac{100}{2} = 50\%$

Miscellaneous questions involving fractions and percentages

Example 1: Finding fraction of an amount

Find $\frac{3}{4}$ of £600, First find $\frac{1}{2}$ = £300, then find $\frac{1}{4}$ (which is half of half) = £150

Therefore $\frac{3}{4}$ = £450 (adding half plus a quarter)

Example 2: Finding a fraction and turning it into a percentage

There are 40 nurses in a small town in Yorkshire. In a particular winter month, 2 nurses have flu.

What is the percentage of nurses that have flu in this winter month?

The fraction of nurses that have flu = $\frac{2}{40}$, by dividing top and bottom numbers by 2 we get $\frac{1}{20}$

To convert 1/20 into a percentage simply multiply 1/20 by 100

= 1/20 X100 =100/20 = 5%

Calculator based questions

You need to remember that percent means out of 100. That is $\frac{1}{100}$. So to find say 42.5% of a number, divide the number by 100 and multiply it by 42.5.

Example: work out 42.5% of £400

We can say that this is the same as (£400 ÷ 100) × 42.5 = 4 × 42.5 = £170

Try working this out with a basic calculator to see if you agree with the answer.

Do the calculations in steps. For example to work out 3.65 + 15×6

Use the rule that you always do multiplication and division before you do addition and subtraction. So to work out 3.65 +15×6, we work out 15×6 first. This gives us 90, then we add 3.65 to 90 to give us 93.65 as the final answer. Note to clear the answer simply click on [C] on the calculator.

Practice Questions involving fractions and percentages

(1) A baby weighs 3 kg at birth. After a few months his weight has now increased by 20%. What is his new weight?

(2) A patient has been asked to increase his exercise routine after being diagnosed with diabetes 2. His baseline number of steps per day is 5000 steps/day. He is asked to increase this to 7500 steps/day in the first instance. What is the percentage increase in steps from his baseline level?

(3) Henry has his annual blood lipid test and it is observed that his Total Cholesterol has decreased from 5.5mmol/l to 5mml/l. What is his percentage decrease in total Cholesterol? Give your answer to the nearest whole number.

(4) Samantha has to increase her medication dosage from 8mg to 10mg. What is the fractional increase?

(5) What is $2\frac{3}{4}$ of 4 litres?

(6) (a) Express 400 ml as a fraction of a litre (b) Convert this fraction to a percentage

(7) What is $\frac{1}{8}$ as a percentage?

(8) What is 35% as a fraction? Give your answer in its simplest form.

(9) A patient loses 20% of his weight due to an illness. His original weight is 90kg. What is his new weight?

(10) John has his Triglycerides monitored. It has reduced from 2.5 mmol/litre to 2.0 mmol/litre. What is the percentage decrease?

Answers to Practice Questions involving fractions and percentages

(1) **Answer:** 3.6kg

Method: Work out 20% of 3kg = $\frac{20}{100} \times 3 = \frac{3}{5} = 0.6$ so his new weight is $3 + 0.6 = 3.6$kg

(2) **Answer:** 50%

Method: From 5000 steps to 7500 steps = an increase of 2500 steps. So the percentage increase from the baseline of 5000 steps is $\frac{2500}{5000} \times 100 = \frac{1}{2} \times 100 = 50\%$

(3) **Answer:** 9%

Method: Decrease in percentage is $\frac{0.5}{5.5} \times 100 = \frac{1}{11} \times 100 = 9\%$ to the nearest whole number.

(4) **Answer:** $\frac{1}{4}$

Method: Increase is 2mg, so the fractional increase from 8mg is $\frac{2}{8} = \frac{1}{4}$

(5) **Answer:** 11 litres

Method: $2\frac{3}{4}$ of $4 = \frac{11}{4} \times 4 = 11$ litres

(6) **Answer** (a) $\frac{2}{5}$ (b) 40%

Method: (a) 400ml as a fraction of 1000ml (1 litre) = $\frac{400}{1000} = \frac{4}{10} = \frac{2}{5}$

(b) Convert $\frac{2}{5}$ into a percentage. So $\frac{2}{5} \times 100 = 40\%$

(7) **Answer:** 12.5%

Method: We know $\frac{1}{4}$ is 25% so $\frac{1}{8}$ is half of 25 = 12.5%

(8) **Answer:** $\frac{7}{20}$

Method: to convert 35% as a fraction we work out $\frac{35}{100}$ and cancel down as much as possible. $\frac{35}{100} = \frac{7}{20}$ (divide top and bottom of $\frac{35}{100}$ by 5)

(9) **Answer**: 72kg

Method: Work out 20% of 90kg. $\frac{20}{100} \times 90 = \frac{1}{5} \times 90 = 18$. We now subtract 18 from 90kg to give us 72kg

(10) **Answer:** 20%

Method: We work out $\frac{0.5}{2.5} \times 100 = \frac{1}{5} \times 100 = 20\%$

Chapter 4   Arithmetic Part 4   Fractions

Simplifying fractions

Reducing a fraction to its lowest terms

Basically you need to find numbers that divide into the top number (numerator) as well as the bottom number (denominator), and then divide them both by the same number (start with 2, if doesn't go then choose 3, then 5, and then the next prime factor e.g. 7, 11, etc.)

Example1: Reduce $\frac{16}{24}$ to its lowest terms.

8 divides exactly into 16 and 24, so in the fraction $\frac{16}{24}$ divide top and bottom by 8. This gives the answer as $\frac{2}{3}$

In case you can't see this straight away, try starting with the number two and work your way numerically upwards using the next prime factor i.e. try 3, then 5 etc. if required

So for the fraction $\frac{16}{24}$ we can start dividing top and bottom by 2 to give us $\frac{8}{12}$, then do the same again as both 8 and 12 are still divisible by 2. This gives us $\frac{4}{6}$ and finally repeating the process once more reduces the fraction to $\frac{2}{3}$ which is the simplest form.

Example 2

Simplify $\frac{9}{12}$ to its lowest terms

In this case we can't divide top and bottom by 2, so we try 3. Since 3 will go into both 9 and 12, we can reduce this to the fraction $\frac{3}{4}$ (since 9 ÷3 =3 and 12 ÷ 3 =4)

Hence, $\frac{9}{12}$ reduces to $\frac{3}{4}$

Example 3: Reduce fraction $\frac{49}{77}$ to its lowest terms. This time we need to spot that 2, 3, 5, does not go into either 49, or 77. Either by trial and error or by spotting the right number we notice 7 goes into both the numerator and the denominator. This reduces

$\frac{49}{77}$ to $\frac{7}{11}$

> **Cancelling down fractions to its simplest form (lowest terms)**
>
> To simplify a fraction to its lowest terms you divide the numerator and the denominator by the same prime factors (2, 3, 5, 7, 11, etc.) to give the equivalent fractions as shown in the examples above

Finding fraction of an amount

Example 1: Find $\frac{2}{5}$ of 25, simply replace the 'of' by X. (times)

So $\frac{2}{5}$ of 25 becomes $\frac{2}{5}$ X 25

To work this out find out 1/5 of 25 and then multiply the answer by 2. So 25 divided by 5, equals 5, then 2 x 5 =10. Hence $\frac{2}{5}$ of 25 =10

> **Example:**
>
> 10 Nurses apply for a certain job vacancy. 4 Nurses are short-listed for an interview. What is the proportion of Nurses that are **not** short listed for the interview? Give your answer as a decimal.
>
> Total number of Nurses applying for this job = 10. Since 4 Nurses are shortlisted, this means 6 are not shortlisted. Hence the proportion that is not shortlisted = 6/10. The answer as a decimal is 0.6

Adding and Subtracting Fractions

This next section will help you revise adding, subtracting, multiplying and dividing fractions together

Consider adding and subtracting fractions together.

When the bottom numbers (denominators) are the same, just add the top numbers together keeping the bottom number the same, likewise for subtraction just subtract the top two numbers.

Example 1: $\frac{2}{5} + \frac{1}{5} = \frac{3}{5}$

Example 2: $\frac{2}{5} - \frac{1}{5} = \frac{1}{5}$

When the denominators are different

Example3: Work out $\frac{1}{2} + \frac{2}{5}$

When the denominators are different, the traditional method of doing this is to find the lowest common denominator. We have to find a number that both 2 and 5 will go into. This is clearly 10.

We can now re-write the fraction with the same common denominator.

To do this we have to ask how did we get the denominator from 2 to 10 for the first part, and likewise for the second part from 5 to 10. The answer is shown below:

$$\frac{1 X 5}{2 X 5} + \frac{2 X 2}{5 X 2} = \frac{5}{10} + \frac{4}{10} = \frac{9}{10}$$

We had to multiply top and bottom by 5 for the first part and top and bottom by 2 for the second part as shown above. We can then add the fraction as we have the same common denominator.

We can however use another very simple strategy that always works. The method is that of crosswise multiplication.

The basic method is to take the fraction sum and do crosswise multiplication as shown by the arrows. In addition, multiply the denominators (bottom numbers) together to get the new denominator.

Example1: $\frac{1}{2} + \frac{2}{5} = \frac{1}{2} \times \frac{2}{5} = \frac{1 X 5 + 2 X 2}{2 X 5} = \frac{5+4}{10} = \frac{9}{10}$

We notice that if we cross multiply as shown we get 1 X 5 and 2 X 2 respectively at the top. To get the bottom number we simply multiply the bottom numbers, 2 and 5 together. So the denominator is 2 X 5=10.

Let us try another example:

Example2: Work out $\frac{3}{7} + \frac{2}{5}$

Using crosswise multiplication and adding rule, as well as multiplying the bottom two numbers we get:

$$\frac{3}{7} \times \frac{2}{5} = \frac{3 X 5 + 7 X 2}{35} = \frac{15+14}{35} = \frac{29}{35}$$

This is a very elegant method which always works

Example 3: Work out $\dfrac{3}{7} - \dfrac{2}{5}$

This is similar to the above except instead of adding we now subtract as shown below.

$$\dfrac{3}{7} \times \dfrac{2}{5} = \dfrac{3X5 - 7X2}{35} = \dfrac{15 - 14}{35} = \dfrac{1}{35}$$

Note: In fact you can use this method when adding or subtracting any fraction that you find difficult. Even if you use this method for simple cases, you will still get the right answer but you may have to cancel down to get the lowest terms for the final answer.

For example we know that $\dfrac{1}{4} + \dfrac{1}{2} = \dfrac{3}{4}$

But if we didn't know and used the method shown we would get $\dfrac{1}{4} \times \dfrac{1}{2} = \dfrac{1X2 + 4X1}{4X2}$
$= \dfrac{2+4}{8} = \dfrac{6}{8} = \dfrac{3}{4}$ (we get this by dividing both the numerator and denominator in $\dfrac{6}{8}$ by 2).
So we get the same answer in the end

Question involving fractions

(1) Find $2\dfrac{3}{4}$ of £64

We first work out 2 X 64 = 128, to work out three quarters of 64 we first work out a half and then add it to a quarter of 64.

Half of £64 is £32

A quarter of £64 (is half of £32) is £16

Hence three quarters of £64 = £32 + £16 = £48

So two and three quarters of £64 = £128 + £48 = £176

Adding and subtracting mixed numbers

We first add or subtract the whole numbers and then the fractional parts.

Ex1: $2\dfrac{2}{5} + 4\dfrac{3}{7}$

Adding the whole numbers we get 6. (Simply add 2 and 4)

Now add the fractional parts to get: $\dfrac{14 + 15}{35} = \dfrac{29}{35}$

So the answer is $6\frac{29}{35}$

Ex2: $4\frac{3}{7} - 2\frac{2}{5}$

Subtract the whole numbers and then the fractional parts, which gives us:

$2\frac{15-14}{35} = 2\frac{1}{35}$

Multiplying Fractions

Multiplying fractions by the traditional method is quite efficient so we will consider only this approach.

Example 1: $\frac{2}{3} \times \frac{5}{7} = \frac{10}{21}$

In this case we simply multiply the top two numbers to get the new numerator and multiply the bottom two numbers together to get the new denominator, as shown above.

Another example will help consolidate this process:

Example 2: $\frac{10}{21} \times \frac{5}{7} = \frac{50}{147}$

(Multiply 10 × 5 to get 50 for the numerator and 21 × 7 to get 147 for the denominator)

Division of Fractions

When dividing fractions we invert the second fraction and multiply as shown.

Think of an obvious example. If we have to divide ½ by ¼ we intuitively know that the answer is 2. The reason for this is that there are 2 quarters in one half. Let us see how this works in practice.

Example 1: $\frac{1}{2} \div \frac{1}{4} = \frac{1}{2} \times \frac{4}{1} = \frac{4}{2} = 2$

Step 1: Re-write fraction as a multiplication sum with the second fraction inverted.

Step 2: Work out the fraction as a normal multiplication

Step 3: Simplify if possible. In this case 4 divided by 2 is 2.

Example 2: $\dfrac{6}{11} \div \dfrac{5}{11} = \dfrac{6}{11} \times \dfrac{11}{5} = \dfrac{66}{55} = \dfrac{6}{5} = 1\dfrac{1}{5}$

Step1: Re-write the fraction inverting the second fraction as shown

Step2: Multiply the top part and the bottom part to get $\dfrac{66}{55}$ as shown.

Step 3: Simplify this by dividing top and bottom by 11 to get $\dfrac{6}{5}$. Now this finally simplifies to $1\dfrac{1}{5}$ as shown.

The following steps are required to convert a mixed number into a fraction. Consider the mixed fraction $2\dfrac{1}{4}$.

Step 1: Multiply the denominator of the fractional part by the whole number and add the numerator. In this case this works out to 2 × 4 + 1 = 9. This now becomes the new numerator.

Step 2: The denominator stays the same as before. Now re-write the new fraction as $\dfrac{9}{4}$. (That is the new numerator ÷ existing denominator)

Let us look at another example. Convert the mixed number, $3\dfrac{3}{7}$ into a fraction.

Step 1: Multiply denominator of fractional part by whole number and add the numerator.

This gives 3 × 7+3 = 24 as the new numerator.

Step2: Re-write fraction as new fraction. This is now the new numerator ÷ existing denominator. This gives us $\dfrac{24}{7}$

Multiplying mixed numbers together

Consider the examples below:

Example: $1\frac{1}{5} \times 1\frac{3}{8}$

The method is simply to convert both mixed numbers into fractions and multiply as shown below:

$$1\frac{1}{5} \times 1\frac{3}{8} = \frac{6}{5} \times \frac{11}{8} = \frac{66}{40} = 1\frac{26}{40} = 1\frac{13}{20}$$

(Notice $\frac{26}{40}$ simplifies to $\frac{13}{20}$)

Dividing mixed numbers together

Example: $1\frac{1}{2} \div 1\frac{1}{4}$

There are two steps required to work out the division of mixed numbers.

Step1: Convert both mixed numbers into fractions as before

Step 2: Multiply the fractions together but invert the second one.

$$1\frac{1}{2} \div 1\frac{1}{4} = \frac{3}{2} \div \frac{5}{4} = \frac{3}{2} \times \frac{4}{5} = \frac{12}{10} = 1\frac{2}{10} = 1\frac{1}{5}$$

More Practice Questions on Fractions and percentages:

(1) Find $\frac{3}{4}$ of 700 millilitres

(2) Find $\frac{4}{5}$ of 650 mcg

(3) Convert $\frac{4}{5}$ to a percentage

(4) What is $\frac{3}{5}$ as a percentage?

(5) Indira and Mukesh decide to get married. Mukesh buys a ring for Indira which is priced at £750. However, he manages to negotiate a 20% discount. How much does Mukesh pay for the ring?

(6) Elizabeth and Gail go for a holiday to Malta for 5 days. They decide to go on an all - inclusive package at a price of £300 each. They manage to book on a last minute deal online which gives them a 30% discount each. How much do they pay in total?

(8) Fiona and Jacob decide to get a small terrace property in Liverpool. Fiona earns £22,500 per annum and Jacob earns £19,500 per annum. They visit their local Building society and are told they can raise a mortgage of 3 times their combined salaries. How much mortgage can they raise between them?

(9) Andy is thinking of purchasing a flat for £95000. He requires a deposit of 15%. How much does he need to have as a deposit?

(10) In a certain Hospital out of 375 Consultants, 12 women and the rest are men. What fraction of the consulting workforce consists of men

(11) What is $\frac{1}{2}$ of £370?

(12) What is 25% of 600 grams?

(13) Sarah buys a dress on ebay for £20. A week later she manages to sell it for £28. What percentage profit does she make?

(14) Macy sells her old car at a 30% loss from the original price. She paid £2300 originally. How much loss did she make?

(15) A sweater is priced at £36. But there is a clearance sale and I can buy it at a quarter of the price. How much do I pay for the sweater?

Answers to Practice Questions on Fractions and Percentages

(1) 525 millilitres

(2) 520 mcg

(3) 80%

(4) 60%

(5) £600

(6) £420 in total

(7) £126,000 Mortgage available

(8) Deposit required is £14,250

(10) $\frac{363}{375}$

(11) £185

(12) 150 grams

(13) 40%

(14) £690 loss

(15) £9

Chapter 5   Proportions and ratios

Although proportion and ratio are related they are not the same thing – see example below for clarification.

Example: In a class there are 15 girls and 10 boys. The **ratio of girls to boys is** 15:10, or 3:2, (divide both 15 and 10 by 5) and the **proportion of girls in the class** is 15 out of 25, $\frac{15}{25}$ **which simplifies to** $\frac{3}{5}$

Questions based on proportions and ratios

Example 1

In a class of 27 pupils, 9 go home for lunch. What is the proportion of pupils in this class that have lunch at school?

Since 9 out of 27 pupils go home, this means 18 pupils have lunch at school.

As a proportion this is 18 out of 27 or $\frac{18}{27}$ which simplifies to $\frac{2}{3}$

Example 2: In a certain work place the ratio of males to females is 2: 3 there are 250 workers altogether. How many of these are male?

Step 1: Find out the total number of parts. You can do this by adding up the ratio parts together. E.g. 2:3 means there are (2+3) = 5 parts altogether. This means 1 part = one fifth of 250 workers = 50 workers.

Since the ratio of male to female is 2:3, there are 2X50 males and 3X50 females

The number of males in this workplace =2X50 = 100

Example 3:

£100 is divided in the ratio 1: 4 how much is the bigger part?

The total number of parts that £100 is divided into is 5 (to find the number of parts simply add the numbers in the ratio, which in this case is 1 and 4)

Clearly, 1 part equals £20 (100 divided by 5), so 4 parts is equal to £80. This is the required bigger part.

Example 4:

As we have seen, sometimes ratios are expressed in ways, which may not be the simplest form. Consider 5:10

(a) You can re-write 5:10 as 1:2 (divide both sides by 5)

(b) 4 : 10 can be re-written as 2 : 5

(c) 8 : 60 can be re-written as 4 : 30 which, simplifies to 2 : 15

(d) 15 : 36 simplifies to 5 : 12 (divide both sides by 3)

Example 5:

A certain medication of 100mg is made up of two solutions. The first solution is 15ml and the second solution is 45ml. (a) What is the ratio of the two solutions, give your answer in its simplest form? (b) What proportion (fraction) does the first solution consists of the total?

>(a) Clearly the ratio of the first solution to the second is 15: 45. However you can simplify this by dividing both sides by 15 to give the ratio as 1: 3 in its simplest form.
>(b) Now we know the total parts of this mixed solution is 4 (adding 1:3). Now the first solution is 1 part of this, so the fraction or proportion of the first solution to the total is $\frac{1}{4}$

Conversions

Conversions are often useful in changing currencies for example from pounds to dollars or euros and vice-versa. It is also useful to convert distances from miles to kilometers or weights from kilograms to pounds and so on.

Basically a conversion involves changing information from one unit of measurement to another. Consider some examples below:

Question based on conversions

Example 1:

I go to France with £150 and convert this into Euros at 1.2 Euros to a pound.

(1) How many Euros do I get? **(2)** I am left with 39 Euros when I get back home. The exchange rate remains the same. How many pounds do I get back?

Method: (1) Since 1 pound = 1.2 Euros, I get 150 X 1.2 =180 Euros in total.

(2) When I get back I change 39 Euros back into pounds. This time I need to divide 39 by 1.2

So 39÷1.2 =32.5. This means I get back £32.50

Example 2: The formula for changing kilometers to miles is given by: $M = \frac{5}{8} \times K$. Use this formula to convert 68 kilometers to miles

Method: substitute **K** with 68 and multiply by $\frac{5}{8}$

This means $M = \frac{5}{8} \times 68$. Using a calculator this comes to 42.5 miles

It is worth reviewing some common Metric and Imperial Conversions

Metric Measures

1000 Millilitres (ml) =1 Litre(l)

100 Centilitres (cl) =1 Litre (l)

10ml =1 cl

1 Centimetre (cm) =10 Millimetres (mm)

1 Metre (m) = 100 cm

1 Kilometre (km) =1000 m

1 Kilogram (kg) =1000 grams (g)

Imperial Measurements

1 foot =12 inches

1 yard =3 feet

1 pound = 16 ounces

1 stone =14 pounds (lb)

1 gallon = 8 pints

1 inch = 2.54 cm (approximately)

Practice Questions on Proportions and Ratios

(1) Mary invites 28 people to her birthday party. 23 of them are girls. What is (a) the proportion of girls in the party? (b) What is the proportion of boys?

(2) Helen cycles to work 3 days out of 5 during a working week. What is the proportion of days she does not cycle to work?

(3) Ahmed has sandwiches 5 times a week for his lunch. For 2 days he has curry. What is the proportion of times he has sandwiches for lunch?

(4) The ratio of sugar to fibre in an orange is 1:7. Assuming an orange weighs 80 grams how many grams of sugar does it contain?

(5) £500 is split between John and James in the ratio of 2:3. How much does James get?

(6) £1200 is divided between 3 people in the ratio of 1:2:3. How much is the largest amount that a person gets?

(7) In 2014 in a particular school 79 people take French out of a total of 690 pupils. What is the proportion of pupils who take French in this school?

(8) I am travelling from Waterloo to Surbiton. The scale on the map is 1: 200000. I measure that on the map this distance is 12cm. How many kilometres is this?

(9) This time I use a map where the scale shown is 1cm = 1 mile. I measure the distance between two places and the distance on the map is 10 cm. How many kilometres is this if you are given that 8 km is equal to 5 miles.

Answers to Practice Questions on Proportions and Ratios

(1) (a) The proportion of girls are $\frac{23}{28}$

(b) The proportion of boys are $\frac{5}{28}$

(2) $\frac{2}{5}$

(3) $\frac{5}{7}$

(4) 10gms

(5) £300

(6) £600

(7) $\frac{79}{690}$

(8) 24km

(9) 16 km

Chapter 6   Formulas

Formula

We have already met some basic formulas when working out various infusion rates. A formula describes the relationship between two or more variables. Consider a formula for working out the BMI (Body Mass Index)

$$BMI = \frac{Body\ Weigt\ (Kg)}{Height^2\ (height\ in\ meters)}$$

Example1: A young adult weighs 63kg and has a height of 1.73m. Work out his BMI to the nearest unit.

Method: We know that $BMI = \frac{Body\ Weigt\ (Kg)}{Height^2\ (height\ in\ meters)} = \frac{63}{1.73^2} = \mathbf{21}$

Example 2:

(1) The formula for working out the distance depends on the speed and time taken in the appropriate units.

D = S×T where D is the distance, S the speed and T is the time.

What is the distance travelled if my speed is 60kmh and I travel for 1hour and 30 minutes.

1 hour 30 minutes corresponds to 1.5 hours so, using the formula, D = 60×1.5 = 90 km

That is, the distance equals 90km

(2) The formula for working out the speed is given as Speed= Distance/Time

That is S = D÷T

Work out the average speed with which I travel, if I cover 100 miles in 2.5 hours.

Since S = D÷T, this means S = 100÷2.5 =40 mph (Notice the units for the first example were in kilometres and units for the second example were in miles

(3) The formula for working out time taken is given by T = D÷S

Calculate the time taken to cover 90 miles if I travel at 60mph?

Time taken, T= D÷S, so T = 90÷60 = 9÷6 =3÷ 2 = 1.5 hours or 1 hour and 30 minutes.

Example 3

The formula for converting the temperature from Celsius to Fahrenheit is given by the formula: $F = \frac{9}{5}C + 32$ (where C is the temperature in degrees Centigrade)

If the temperature is 10 degrees Celsius then what is the equivalent in temperature in Fahrenheit?

Using the formula $F = \frac{9}{5}C + 32$, and substituting 10 in place of C, we have $F = \frac{9}{5} \times 10 + 32 = \frac{90}{5} + 32 = 18 + 32 = 50$. Hence, 10 degrees centigrade = 50 degrees Fahrenheit

(**Explanation of working out above**: Remember we multiply and divide before adding and subtracting) There are no brackets to worry about. When working out $\frac{9}{5} \times 10 + 32$, multiply 9 by 10 to get 90, divide this by 5 to get 18, finally add 18 and 32 together to get 50

Example 3: Convert 68 degrees Fahrenheit to degrees Celsius. The formula for converting the temperature from Fahrenheit to Celsius is given by:

$C = \frac{5}{9}(F - 32)$. To change 68 degrees Fahrenheit to degrees Celsius we can substitute for F in the formula $C = \frac{5}{9}(F - 32)$., $C = C = \frac{5}{9}(68 - 32)$. $= 5 \times 36/9 = 5 \times 4 = 20$

Hence, 68 degrees Fahrenheit = 20 degrees Celsius

(**Explanation of the working out above**: Using BIDMAS we work out the bracket first. This gives us 68-32 =36. We now divide this by 9 and multiply by 5. Clearly 36÷9 =4 and finally 5X4 =20)

Practice Questions on Formulas

(1) You are given that Speed = $\frac{\text{Distance}}{\text{Time}}$. Calculate my speed in m.p.h if I travel 25 miles in half an hour.

(2) John is a travelling salesman. He gets expenses at 25p for every mile he covers and £25 to cover his lunch and dinner every day. The formula the company uses to work out his expenses for a given number of days is given by E = 0.25m + 25d (where m is the number of miles covered and d is the number of days he has been travelling). One week he travels 360 miles in 4 days. How much will he receive in expenses altogether for this week?

(3) Whilst she is in France Miranda wants to convert the number of kilometres she has covered into miles. She notes the formula for converting kilometres into miles is given by M = $\frac{5}{8}$ X K. Assuming she covers 480 km how many miles is this?

(4) The formula for converting degrees centigrade into Fahrenheit is given by the formula F= $\frac{9}{5}$C +32. What is the temperature in Fahrenheit if it is 25 degrees centigrade?

(5) Joe has been told that he needs to reduce his body mass index to below 25 as he is presently a bit overweight. He presently weighs 90kg and is 1.8m tall. He decides to lose 10kg in the next 3 months. The formula for working out the body mass index is given by:

BMI = Weight ÷ $height^2$

- (c) What is his present BMI?
- (d) What will be his BMI after losing 10Kg, give the answer to one decimal place?
- (e) Does he achieve his goals?

Answers to Practice Questions on Formulas

(1) 50 mph

(2) E = 0.25m + 25d, so E = 0.25×360+ 25×4 = £190

(3) 300 miles

(4) 77°F

(5) (a) BMI = 27.8 (to one decimal place)

　　(b) After losing 10Kg, Joes's BMI = 24.7 (to one decimal place)

　　(c) Yes

Chapter 7: Data Interpretation

Mean, Median, Mode and Range

First consider the different types of 'averages'.

That is Mean, Median, Mode and Range (You can try to remember these as: MMMR)

Mean: The sum of the numbers in a data set divided by the number of values in the Set

Median: The middle number of a data set when listed in order

Mode: The most frequently occurring number or numbers in a data set

Range: The difference between the highest and the smallest numbers in a data set

Example 1:
Find the mean value of the following data set:
2, 7, 1, 1, 7, 8, 9

Method: Find the sum first
2 + 7 + 1 + 1 + 7 + 8 + 9 = 35
Now divide this total by 7, since this is the total number of numbers
So, 35/7 = 5
Hence, the mean value of this data set is 5

Example 2:
Find the median of 3, 7, 1, 8, and 6

Method: First re-order from smallest to biggest, re-writing the numbers we have: 1, 3, 6, 7, 8
Clearly the middle number is 6.
Hence, the median is 6

Example 3:
Find the median of 3, 6, 7, 1, 8 and 5

Method
First re-arrange to get 1, 3, 5, 6, 7, 8
Notice, in this case the middle number is between 5 & 6
So the median is (5 + 6)/2 = 5.5

Example 4:
Find the Range of the data set 3, 5, 7, 1, 8, and 11

Method: Find the difference between the biggest and smallest numbers
So the Range = 11 – 1 = 10

Example 5:
Find the Mode of the following numbers:
1, 4, 4, 4, 7, 8, 9, 9, 11, 12

Method: Find the most frequently occurring number. The most frequently occurring number is 4.
Hence the Mode is 4

Example 6:
Find the mode of 1, 3, 3, 3, 3 5, 5, 5, 5, 8, 8, 9

Method: As before find the most frequently occurring number(s).
Clearly there are two modes here. Both '3' and '5' occur most frequently, the same number of times, so we say this is a bi-modal distribution. That is, a distribution with two modes, namely 3 and 5

Pie Charts

When data is represented in a circle this is called a pie chart. Basically you need to remember that a full circle or 360 degrees represents all the data (or 100% of the data). Half a circle or 180 degrees represents half the data (or 50% of the data), and similarly 25% of the data is represented by 90 degrees or a quarter of a circle. Essentially, each sector or slice of the pie chart shows the proportion of the total data in that category.

Example 1:

The pie chart below shows the percentage of applicants who got different grades in a psychometric aptitude test when applying for a job in a particular company. The requirement to be short listed for a second interview was to pass with high marks. If 140 applicants took this test how many of them were short listed?

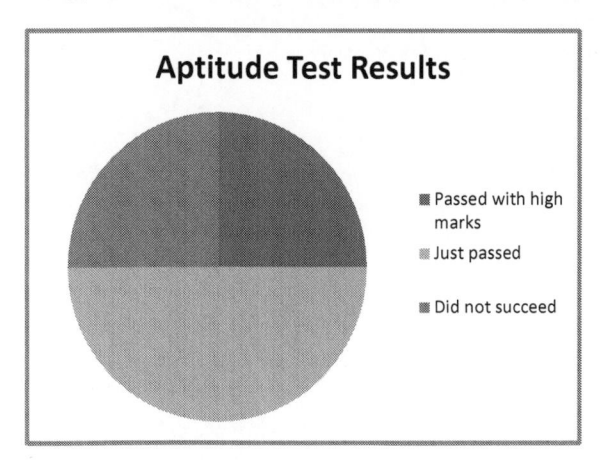

Aptitude Test Results

- Passed with high marks
- Just passed
- Did not succeed

Method: As illustrated the results in this aptitude test for this particular company show that 25% got the required 'high marks' to be short listed for a second interview. Since a quarter of a circle corresponds to 25%. This means a quarter of the 140 applicants attained this which corresponds to 35 people.

Example 2:

The destination of 120 pupils who leave year 11 in School B in 2012 is represented in the pie chart below. The numbers outside the sectors represent the number of pupils

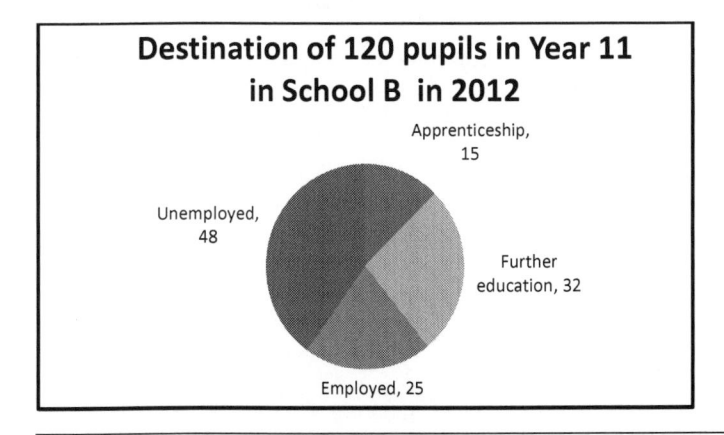

Destination of 120 pupils in Year 11 in School B in 2012

- Apprenticeship, 15
- Unemployed, 48
- Further education, 32
- Employed, 25

(1) What is the percentage of pupils who are unemployed?

Method:

The number of pupils out of 120 that are unemployed is 48. So the percentage of pupils who are unemployed is $\frac{48}{120} \times 100 = \frac{4800}{120} = \frac{480}{12} = 40\%$

(2) What fraction of pupils go on to Further Education?

Method:

The fraction of pupils that go on to further education is $\frac{32}{120} = \frac{8}{30} = \frac{4}{15}$, the fraction representing this in its simplest form is $\frac{4}{15}$

(3) What percentage of pupils is either employed or in apprenticeships? Give your answer to one decimal place?

Method:

Total number of pupils who are either in employment or apprenticeships = 25+15 =40, hence the percentage is $\frac{40}{120} \times 100 = \frac{4}{12} \times 100 = \frac{1}{3} \times 100 = 33.3\%$

Bar charts

Bar charts can be represented in columns or as horizontal bars. They can be either simple bar charts that show frequencies associated with data values or they can be multiple bar charts to allow for comparisons between data sets as shown below. The examples below illustrate some of the ways bar charts can be used to represent data.

Example 1: In a cosmetics shop the number of items that were sold for four top brands over a one month period were recorded as shown in the bar chart below.

(1) Which brand had the highest sales? **You can see from the column bar chart below that Brand D had the highest sales as 40 items of this brand were sold during one month, which is higher than any other brand**

(2) What was the proportion of sales for Brand D compared to the total? Give your answer as a fraction in its lowest terms. **The number of Brand A items sold were 20, Brand B were 35 and Brand C were 25 and as we saw earlier 40 items of Brand D were sold. This means the total number of cosmetic items sold during this one month period = 120. Since 40 items belonged to Brand D, compared to the total this is $\frac{40}{120}$ which simplifies to $\frac{1}{3}$**

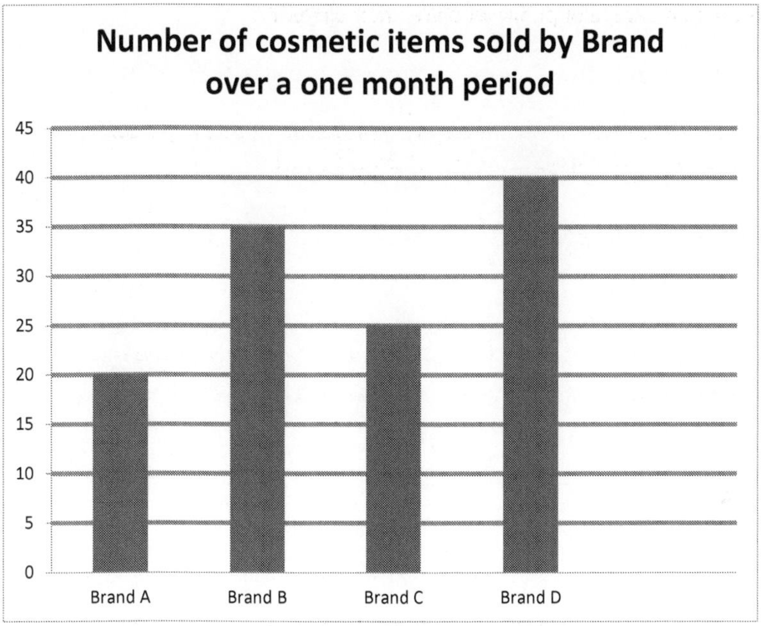
Number of cosmetic items sold by Brand over a one month period
45
40
35
30
25
20
15
10
5
0
Brand A
Brand B
Brand C
Brand D

Example 2:

The bar chart below shows the amount of time in hours John, Bob and Bill spend surfing the web at weekends. What is the mean time per boy that is spent surfing the web at the weekend?

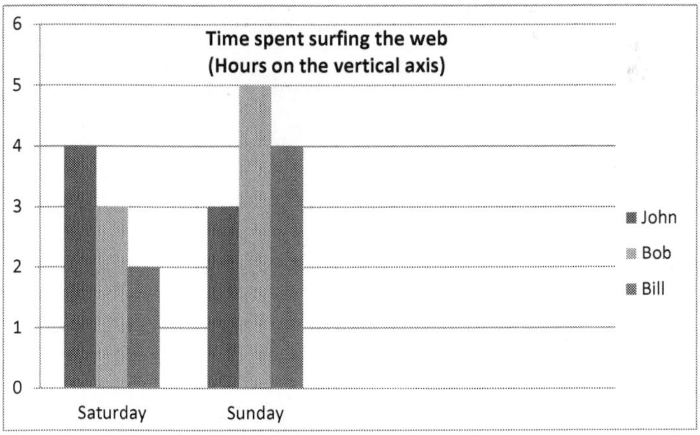
Time spent surfing the web
(Hours on the vertical axis)
6
5
4
3
2
1
0
Saturday
Sunday
John
Bob
Bill

Method: John spends 4 hours on Saturday and 3 hours on a Sunday: a total of 7 hours

Bob spends a total of 3 hours on Saturday and 5 hours on Sunday: a total of 8 hours

Similarly, Bill spends a total of 2 + 4 = 6 hours on a weekend

Total time spent surfing between the 3 boys on a week end is 7+ 8 + 6 =21hours

Hence the mean time spent per boy is 21 ÷ 3 =7 hours

Line graph

A line graph is a way to represent two sets of related data. **It is often used to show trends**

Example 1: The data below shows the percentage of patients in a certain hospital who were admitted with heart attacks from 2005 to 2010. This data is shown in the table below. However, the same data can be shown as a line graph that follows.

Year	2005	2006	2007	2008	2009	2010
% of patients admitted with Heart attacks	26%	35%	45%	37%	48%	32%

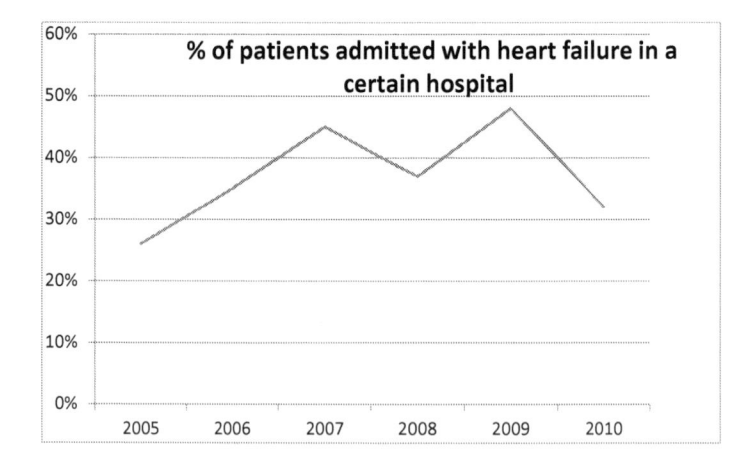

% of patients admitted with heart failure in a certain hospital

Year	%
2005	26%
2006	35%
2007	45%
2008	37%
2009	48%
2010	32%

Practice questions on Data Interpretation

(1) What is mean of 3, 7, 8, 2, 9 and 1?

(2) Find the median of 5, 7, 2, 8, and 4

(3) Find the range of the data set 2, 6, 9, 1, 4, and 15

(4) In the Pie chart below what fraction of students did not succeed?

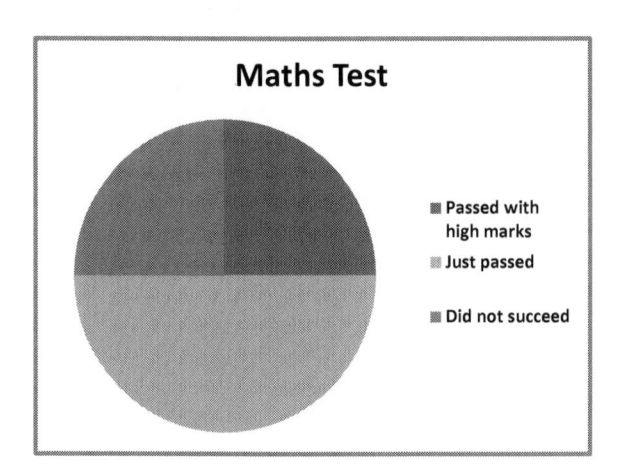

Maths Test
- Passed with high marks
- Just passed
- Did not succeed

(5) The bar chart below shows the number of nurses employed in four hospitals. How many Nurses are employed there in Hospital D?

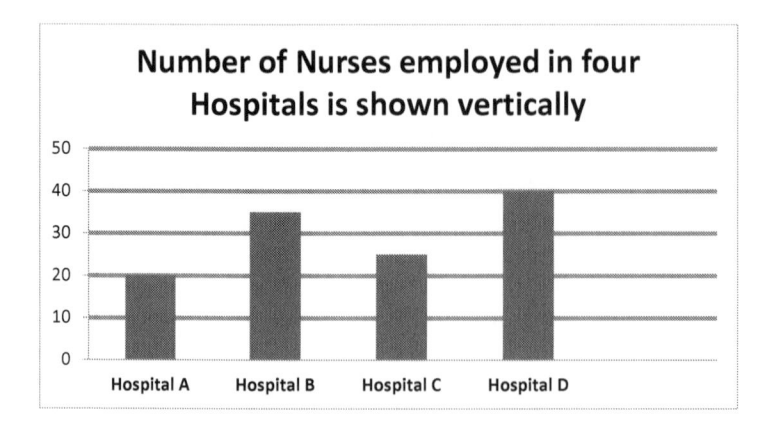

Number of Nurses employed in four Hospitals is shown vertically

Hospital A	Hospital B	Hospital C	Hospital D
20	35	25	40

(6) The bar chart below shows the amount of additional tuition time in hours that Samantha, Joanna and Yasmin spend per week in Maths

and English. (a) How many hours of tuition per week does Samantha spend in a week in both subjects? (b) What is mean tuition time spent by the three students in maths?

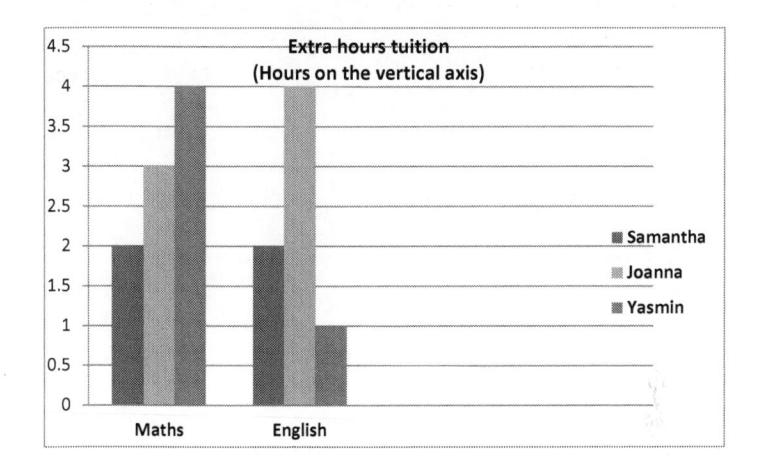

Extra hours tuition
(Hours on the vertical axis)

Bar chart showing Maths: Samantha 2, Joanna 3, Yasmin 4; English: Samantha 2, Joanna 4, Yasmin 1.

Answers to Practice Questions on Data Interpretation

(1) 5

(2) 5

(3) 14

(4) $\frac{1}{2}$ or 0.5

(5) 40

(6) (a) Samantha spends a total of 4 hours in tuition in a week

   (b) 3 hours

Mock Tests

On the next page you will find 4 Mock Tests with detailed answers at the end of each test. **Try to complete the test in 25 minutes, you should aim to get 16 out of 20 questions right in each test**. Do not worry if you do not make it the first time round. You can go back to the examples in the questions you found difficult and repeat the tests. Good luck with your actual tests.

Tip: Remember some basics shown below:

Volume measures

1 litre(l) = 1000 Millilitres (ml)

Mass (weight) measures

1 Kilogram (kg) =1000 grams (g)

1 Gram (g) = 1000 milligrams (mg)

1 Milligram (mg) = 1000 micrograms (mcg)

1 Microgram (mcg) = 1000 Nano grams (ng)

Most frequently used abbreviations that you might find useful:

o.d – once daily

b.d. – Twice daily

t.d.s. - Three times daily

q.d.s. – Four times daily

a.c - Before meals

p.c – After meals

In most cases you can work the answers to the questions in these tests without using any special formula. However, do not forget to <u>double check your answers.</u>

Mock Test 1 - 25 Minutes   No Calculators Allowed

(1) Convert 25grams to milligrams

(2) Convert 2.67grams to milligrams

(3) Convert 750mg to g

(4) Convert 1020 mcg to mg

(5) Convert 1.25g to mcg

(6) Convert 140 ml to litres

(7) Convert 2450ml to litres

(8) A patient needs 500mg of a particular tablet to be taken over a day. The tablets come in 125mg dose. How many tablets should the patient take over a day?

(9) Karim is prescribed 750mg of a particular drug to be taken as a solution. The solution contains 125mg of the drug per 25ml. How many ml should Karim take?

(10) Jenna been prescribed 80mg of propranolol to be taken twice a day. The tablets she has been given are 20mg each. How many tablets does Jenna have to take in total per day?

(11) A patient is prescribed 750 mg of this liquid medicine per day. This particular solution comes in 50 ml for every 125 mg. How many ml of this solution is required in a given day?

(12) Mary has been prescribed a certain drug 3mg/kg/day to be taken in three divided doses. Anna weighs 60Kg. (a) Calculate her total daily dose (b) Work out her single dose.

(13) Michael has been prescribed a certain drug 4mg/kg/day to be taken in two divided doses. Michael weighs 74Kg. (a) Calculate his total daily dose (b) Work out his single dose.

(14) Philip is advised to increase his Statins from 20mg to 40 mg per day. What is the percentage increase?

(15) A patient is asked to cut down on sugar and exercise more in order to reduce his weight for his given height. His initial weight is 96kg. He manages to lose 12kg. What percentage loss does this patient achieve?

(16) A patient is administered 800ml over 5 hours. How many ml (millilitres) has been administered over 2 hours?

(17) A patient has been prescribed to take 1200 ml of a certain fluid. The patient has taken 40%. How many ml of fluid has he still to take?

(18) Convert 2.5 mcg to ng (Nano grams)

(19) A patient takes 25% of his required daily dose. What fraction of the dose still remains to be taken?

(20) The stock tablets you have are 400 mcg. A patient has been prescribed 1.6mg per day. How many tablets does the patient need to be given on a day?

Answers to Mock Test 1

(1) Answer: 25000mg

Method: There are 1000mg in each gram so in 25g there are: 25×1000 =25000mg

(2) Answer: 2670mg

Method: As above. 2.67×1000 =2670mg

(3) Answer: 0.75g

Method: Since each gram has 1000 mg this time we divide 750 by 1000. 750÷1000 = 0.75g

(4) Answer: 1.02mg

Method: Divide 1020 by 1000. So 1020÷1000 = 1.02mg

(5) Answer: 1250000 mcg

Method: There are 1000mg in one gram and 1000mcg in one mg so we need to work out 1.25×1000×1000 = 1250×1000 = 1250000mcg

(6) Answer: 0.14 litres

Method: There are 1000ml in 1litre. So we need to work out 140÷1000=0.14 litres

(7) Answer: 2.45 litres

Method: Divide 2450 by 1000 to get 2.45 litres

(8) Answer: 4 tablets

Method: Total dose =500mg, each tablet = 125mg so we need 500÷125 =4

(9) Answer: 150ml

Method: 25 ml has 125mg. So 750mg has $\frac{750}{125}$ ×25 = 6×25 = 150ml

(10) Answer: 8 tablets

Method: 80mg twice a day = 160mg. Each tablet is 20mg so Jenna needs 160÷20 = 8 tablets per day

(11) Answer: 300ml

Method: 125mg contained in 50ml of solution. So 750mg needs: $\frac{750}{125}$×50 = 6×50 = 300ml

(12) Answer: (a) 180mg in total (b) 60mg per dose

Method: (a) Since the prescribed drug is 3mg/kg/day and she weighs 60kg we need to work out 60×3 =180mg.(b) Divided by three equal doses means 180÷3 =60mg/dose

(13) Answer: (a) 296mg (b) 148mg

Method: (a) As the previous question work out 4×74 = 296mg in total. Then work out 296÷2 = 148mg per single dose.

(14) Answer: 100%

Method: Dose increase is 20mg from a base of 20mg. So percentage increase is $\frac{20}{20}$×100 = 100%

(15) Answer: 12.5%

Method: $\frac{12}{96}$×100 = $\frac{1}{8}$×100 = $\frac{1}{4}$×50 = $\frac{1}{2}$×25 = 12.5%

(16) Answer: 320ml

Method: The amount that has been administered in 2hours is $\frac{2}{5}$×800 = 2×160=320ml

(17) Answer: 720ml

Method: He has 60% left to take, So 60% of 1200ml is $\frac{60}{100}$×1200 =60×12 =720ml

(18) Answer: 2500 Nano grams

Method: There are 1000 Nano grams in one micro gram. So 2.5mcg = 2.5×1000 = 2500 Nano Grams

(19)Answer: $\frac{3}{4}$ remains

Method: He has taken 25% or $\frac{1}{4}$ of his dose. So $\frac{3}{4}$ remains

(20) Answer: 4 tablets

Method: 1.6mg = 1600mcg. Since each tablet is 400mcg. Number of tablets required is $\frac{1600}{400}$ = 4 tablets

Mock Test 2 - 25 Minutes No Calculators Allowed

(1) Convert 2.35grams to micrograms

(2) Convert 2050 mcg to mg

(3) A patient needs 600mg of a tablet to be taken over a day. The tablets come in 150mg dose. How many tablets should the patient take over a day?

(4) Joanna is prescribed 900mg of a particular drug to be taken as a solution. The solution contains 150mg of the drug per 30 ml. How many ml should Joanna take?

(5) A patient has been advised to take 100mcg of Levothyroxine per day for her hypothyroidism. (a) How many mcg of Levothyroxine does this patient consume over 21 days? (b) How many mg is this equivalent to over 21 days?

(6) A patient is prescribed 600 mg of this liquid medicine per day. This particular solution comes in 40 ml for every 150 mg. How many ml of this solution is required in a given day?

(7) A hospital doctor requests that a patient receives 2 litres of normal Saline over the next 5 hours. What is the infusion rate in ml/hour (milli-litres per hour)?

(8) A patient is prescribed 0.5 litres of normal Saline over the next two hours. What is the infusion drop rate per minute if the drop rate is 30?

Hint: The formula to work out the Infusion Rate in drops per minute is given by:

$$\frac{Volume\ required\ (ml)}{hours} \times \frac{drop\ factor}{60}$$

(9) This time a patient is prescribed 0.8 litres of normal Saline over the next four hours. What is the infusion drop rate per minute if the drop rate is 24?

(10) Dextrose 5% is infused at a rate of 60ml/hour. How much dextrose is infused after 6 hours and 30 minutes?

(11) A certain solution contains a drug which has a strength of 0.3% w/v. How many mg of this drug are there in 40ml of this solution?

(12) A solution of Sodium Chloride has a concentration of 0.4% w/v. How many grams of Sodium Chloride are there in this 0.75 litres of Saline solution?

(13) 1.2 liters of a particular fluid is given at an infusion rate of 200 ml/hour. How long will the infusion last in hours?

(14) A patient has to have 0.5mg of a certain tablet 4 times a day with an interval of 4 hours before the next dose. Assuming the first dose is given at 8.30am. When is the last dose given? Give your answer using the 24 hour clock

(15) A patient receives 0.6 liters of dextrose over 4 hours. What is the infusion rate in ml/hour?

(16) A certain medication of 150mg is made up of two solutions. The first solution is 25ml and the second solution is 75ml. What is the ratio of the two solutions, give your answer in its simplest form?

(17) John has to increase her medication dosage from 5mg to 6.5mg. What is the percentage increase in his dose?

(18) A patient who is on 2500mcg of clonazepam per day is asked to gradually reduce his intake. He is asked to reduce his intake by 20%. The tablets the patient is taking comes in 500mcg tablets. How many tablets should he be taking during his reduction phase?

(19) Amanda has to increase her dosage of a tablet from 60 mcg to 75mcg. What is the percentage increase?

(20) Mr. Patel is prescribed 960mg of a particular drug to be taken as a solution. The solution contains 120mg of the drug per 30ml. How many ml should Mr. Patel take?

Answers for Mock Test 2

(1) Answer: 2350000 mcg

Method: 2.35 grams has 2.35×1000 mg = 2350×1000 mcg =2350000 mcg

(2) Answer: 2.05mg

Method: This time we divide 2050 by 1000 to convert mcg to mg. So 2050÷1000 = 2.05mg

(3) Answer: 4 tablets per day

Method: Patient needs 600mg. Tablet dose is 150mg. So number of tablets required is 600÷150 = 4 tablets

(4) Answer: 180ml

Method: 30ml contains 150mg. Joanna needs 900mg which is equal to $\frac{900}{150} \times 30 = 6 \times 30 = 180$ ml

(5) Answer: (a) 2100mcg (b) 2.1mg

Method: (a) A patient takes 100mcg/day. So over 21 days this equals 21×100=2100mcg (b) to convert 2100mcg to mg we divide 2100 by 1000. 2100÷1000 = 2.1mg

(6) Answer: 160ml

Method: Since 40ml has 150mg this means 600mg has: $\frac{600}{150} \times 40$ =160ml

(7) Answer: 400ml/hour

Method: 2 liters = 2000 ml. This means 2000 ml of normal Saline has to be infused over 4 hours. So the infusion rate in ml/hour = 2000÷5 = 400ml/hour

The basic formula to remember in this case is **Infusion Rate (ml/hour) = Volume in ml ÷ Time (hours)**

(8) Answer: 125 drops/min

Method: Infusion drop rate(ml)/min = $\frac{500(ml)}{2(hours)} \times \frac{30(drop\ factor)}{60} = 125$

(9) Answer: 80 drops/min

Method: Infusion drop rate(ml)/min = $\frac{800(ml)}{4(hours)} \times \frac{24(drop\ factor)}{60} = 80$

(10) Answer: 390 ml

Method: Volume = Rate (ml/hour) × total running time (hours), so Volume = 60×6.5 (Since 6hours 30 minutes = 6.5 hours). 60×6.5 = 360 + 30 = 390ml

(11) Answer: 120mg

Method: 0.3% means 0.3g/100ml. Now we know that 0.3g = 0.3×1000 = 300mg. This means if 100 ml has 300mg, so 40ml has $\frac{40}{100}$ × 300mg = 120mg of this drug.

(12) Answer: 3g

Method: 0.4% w/v means 0.4g/100ml. So 0.75 litres (750ml) has $\frac{750}{100}$×0.4 g = 7.5×0.4 = 3g

(13) Answer: 6 hours

Method: Infusion times = $\frac{Volume\ to\ be\ infused\ (ml)}{Rate\ (ml\ per\ hour)} = \frac{1200\ (ml)}{200\ (ml\ per\ hour)}$ = 6hours

(14) Answer: 2030

Method: First dose at 8.30 (so last dose is 3×4 = 12hours later (It is 3× and not 4× as the first dose has already been given. Hence the last dose is at 2030

(15) Answer: 150ml/hour

Method: Basic infusion rate = $\frac{volume(ml)}{Time(hrs)} = \frac{600(ml)}{4(hrs)}$ = 150ml/hour

(16) Answer: 1: 3 in its simplest form

Method: The ratio of the two solutions is 25:75 which simplifies to 1:3 (divide both 25 &75 in the first ratio by 25)

(17) Answer: 30%

Method: Increase in dose =1.5mg. So percentage increase is $\frac{1.5}{5}$×100 =1.5×20 =30%

(18) Answer: 4 tablets

Method: Reduction of 20% from 2500 is $\frac{20}{100} \times 2500 = 20 \times 25 = 500$mcg. So his new intake is 2500 − 500 = 2000mcg. Since each tablet is 500mcg the patient now needs to take 2000÷500 = 4 tablets

(19) Answer: 25%

Method: Increase is 15mcg from 60mcg. So the percentage increase is $\frac{15}{60} \times 100 = \frac{1}{4} \times 100 = 25\%$

(20) Answer: 240ml

Method: Since there is 120mg of the drug in 30ml, this means we need to work out $\frac{960}{120} \times 30 = 8 \times 30 = 240$ml

Mock Test 3 - 25 Minutes   No Calculators Allowed

(1) A solution contains 30mg of a drug in 12ml. What is the concentration in mg/ml?

(2) A syringe contains 16mg of morphine in 4ml. What is the concentration in mg/ml

(3) Convert 5.65g to mg

(4) Convert 445 ml to litres

(5) A patient has been prescribed 0.09mg of a particular drug. The stock tablets you have are 30mcg. How many tablets should this patient have?

(6) The TTD (Total daily dose) is 600mg. The Stock tablets are 150mg and have to be given twice a day. How many tablets are given once?

(7) 0.9mg of a drug is prescribed. The stock is 0.3mg in 4ml. What volume has to be administered?

(8) What is 40% of 700mcg in mg?

(9) David is prescribed 1.2mg/kg/dose of a certain drug. David weighs 85kg. How many mg will he need per dose?

(10) Michelle has been prescribed erythromycin, 35mg/kg/dose. Her weight is 62kg. How many grams of drug does each dose constitute?

(11) 0.6 litres of a solution is given at the rate of 200ml/hour. The infusion starts at 1330. What time will it end? Give your answer in 24 hour clock.

(12) A patient receives 60ml of Saline in 45 minutes. What is the infusion rate in ml/hour?

(13) Convert 10mcg/minute to mg/hour

(14) The daily prophylactic dose of a certain drug for an adult is between 40-60mg/kg of body weight. What is the maximum dose in grams that can be given to patient weighing 65kg?

(15) A child is to receive 1.2 litres of fluid over 8 hours. What is the infusion rate in drops/minute if the drop factor is 20?

(16) 250ml of blood is to be infused over 2hours and 30minutes. What is the infusion rate in drops/minute if the drop factor is 30?

(17) A patient has been prescribed Cephalothin, 30mg/kg/dose tds (three times a day). The patient weighs 88kg. How many g of this tablet does the patient consume in a day?

(18) A patient is asked to increase her amitriptyline dose from 50mg to 80 mg per day. What percentage increase is this?

(19) Convert 12000000 mcg to Kilograms

(20) A medication of 250mg is made up of three solutions. The first solution is 50ml and the second solution is 75ml and the third solution is 100ml. What is the ratio of these three solutions, give your answer in its simplest form?

Answers to Mock Test 3

(1) Answer: 2.5mg/ml

Method: Since there are 30mg in 12ml then 1ml has $\frac{30}{12} = \frac{15}{6} = 2.5\text{mg}$

(2) Answer: 4mg/ml

Method: Since there are 16mg in 4ml then 1ml has $\frac{16}{4} = 4\text{mg}$

(3) Answer: 5650mg

Method: Multiply 5.65 by 1000 to convert g to mg. We get 5.65×1000 = 5650mg

(4) Answer: 0.445 litres

Method: Divide 445 ml by 1000 to convert ml to litres. We get 445÷1000 = 0.445 litres

(5) Answer: 3 tablets

Method: 0.09mg = 0.09×1000 mcg = 90mcg. Since the tablets come in 30mcg the patient needs to have 90÷30 = 3 tablets

(6) Answer: 2 tablets

Method: TTD is 600mg given twice a day. This means one dose is 300mg. But the tablets are 150mg each so the patient needs 300÷150 = 2 tablets/dose

(7) Answer: 12ml

Method: 4ml contains 0.3mg of the prescribed drug. So 0.9mg has to be three times 4ml. 3×4 =12ml

(8) Answer: 0.28mg

Method: 40% of 700mcg is $\frac{40}{100}$×700= 40×7 =280mcg = 0.28mg

(9) Answer: 102mg

Method: Since David weighs 85kg the dose required is 1.2×85 = 102mg

(10) Answer: 2.17g

Method: Michelle needs 35×62 =2170mg = 2.17g

(11) Answer: 1630

Method: Since the infusion rate is 200ml/hour for 0.6 litres the time taken is: $\frac{600}{200}$ = 3 hours. If the infusion starts at 1330 it will end at 1630.

(12) Answer: 80ml/hour

Method: 60ml of Saline is infused over 45miutes is. So every 15minutes, 20ml is infused hence every 60 minutes (1 hour) 20×4 =80ml is infused. So the infusion rate is 80ml/hour. **Alternate method:** Infusion Rate $=\frac{Volume\ (ml)}{Time\ (hours)}=\frac{60}{\frac{3}{4}}=60\times\frac{4}{3}=20\times 4=80$ml/hour

(13) Answer: 0.6mg/hour

Method: 10mcg/minute =600mcg per hour = 600÷1000 mg/hour = 0.6mg/hour

(14) Answer: Maximum dose is 3.9grams

Method: Maximum dose is 60×65 =3900mg =3900÷1000 g = 3.9grams

(15) Answer: 50 drops/minute

Method: Infusion Rate in drops per minute $=\frac{Volume\ required\ (ml)}{hours}\times\frac{drop\ factor}{60}$

So infusion rate = = $\frac{1200\ (ml)}{8}\times\frac{20}{60}=\frac{1200}{8}\times\frac{1}{3}=\frac{400}{8}$ =50 drops/minute

(16) Answer: 50 drops/minute

Method: Infusion Rate in drops per minute $=\frac{Volume\ required\ (ml)}{hours}\times\frac{drop\ factor}{60}$

So infusion rate = = $\frac{250\ (ml)}{2.5}\times\frac{30}{60}=\frac{250}{2.5}\times\frac{1}{2}=\frac{250}{5}$ =50 drops/minute

(17) Answer: 7.92g/day

Method: Patient takes 3 times a day. =90mg/kg/day. Since the patient weighs 88kg this is equivalent to 90×88mg = 7920mg =7920÷1000 g = 7.92g/day

(18) Answer: 60%

Method: Increase is 30mg from a base of 50mg. So percentage increase is $\frac{30}{50} \times 100 = 60\%$

µ**(19) Answer**: 0.012kg

Method: 12000000mcg = 12000000÷1000 mg = 12000mg = 12g = 12÷1000kg = 0.012kg

(20) Answer: 2:3:4

Method: The ratio of the three solutions is 50:75:100 = 2:3:4 (divide each bit of the former ratio by 25)

Mock Test 4 - 25 Minutes   No Calculators Allowed

(1) A patient is prescribed 720 ml over 8 hours. How many ml remain to be given after 2 hours?

(2) Mary has a daily fluid allowance of 1600ml. So far Mary has taken 40% of her allowance. How many ml remain to be taken by Mary?

(3) A patient has been prescribed 75 milligrams of a certain drug. The stock dose is 25mg/10ml. What volume does the patient need?

(4) A patient has been prescribed 12.5mg of Drug A. The stock is available as 2.5mg tablet. How many tablets does this patient need to take?

(5) The waist circumference of a certain patient is 40inches. After 3 months of good diet and exercise the waistline reduces to 38 inches. What is the percentage reduction in this patient's waistline?

(6) Joseph is prescribed 900 mg of this liquid medicine per day. This particular solution comes in 50 ml for every 150 mg. How many ml of this solution is required in a given day?

(7) Dextrose 5% is infused at a rate of 40ml/hour. How much dextrose is infused after 5 hours and 45 minutes?

(8) Convert 3450 mcg to mg

(9) Fatima has been prescribed a certain drug 2.5mg/kg/day to be taken in two divided doses. Fatima weighs 58Kg. (a) Calculate her total daily dose (b) Work out her single dose.

(10) A patient is prescribed 0.6 litres of normal Saline over the next 5 hours. What is the infusion drop rate per minute if the drop rate is 25?

(11) A patient is prescribed 3 mg of Prednisolone daily. The stock is available in 1mg. How many tablets will the patient take in 30 days?

(12) 0.45 litres of a solution is given at the rate of 150 ml/hour. The infusion starts at 1450. What time will it end? Give your answer in 24 hour clock.

(13) 300ml of blood is to be infused over 2hours and 30 minutes. What is the infusion rate in drops/minute if the drop factor is 30?

(14) A Cardiac Nurse is giving advice to a patient about cholesterol lipid levels. She tells a patient that her ratio of Total Cholesterol to HDL (High density lipoproteins) should ideally be 4 or less. The patient has a Total Cholesterol of 6mmol/L and an HDL of 1.5mmol/L. Does this patient meet the criteria set out by the nurse?
(N.B. mmol/L stands for millimoles per litre)

(15) 600 mg of a drug in powder is reconstituted with 5.5 ml of sterile water for an injection. The displacement volume is 0.5ml. What volume needs to be administered for a dose of 200mg?

(16) A patient receives 1.2 litres of fluid over 8 hours. What is the infusion rate in drops/minute if the drop factor is 30.

(17) Convert 0.75g to mcg

(18) A patient increases her amitriptyline dose from 50mg to 80mg. What is the percentage increase?

(19) A patient has to increase his Levothyroxine dose from 50mg to 75mg. What percentage does this constitute?

(20) A patient has been prescribed a certain drug, 20mcg/kg/dose, qds (four times a day). The patient weighs 90kg. How many mg of this tablet does the patient consume in a day?

Answers to Mock Test 4

(1) Answer: 560ml

Method: The patient consumes 720÷8 =90ml/hour. So in two hours 160ml is given. This means 720 – 180 = 540ml remain

(2) Answer: 960ml

Method: 40% of 1600ml =$\frac{40}{100}$ ×1600 =40×16 =640ml. So the amount of fluid that remains to be taken by Mary is 1600 – 640 = 960ml

(3) Answer: 30ml

Method: If 25mg is contained in 10ml then 75mg needs $\frac{75}{25}$ ×10 =3×10 =30ml

(4) Answer: 5 tablets

Method: We simply divide 12.5 by 2.5 to find the number of tablets. This gives us $\frac{12.5}{2.5}$ = 5. Check 5×2.5 =12.5

(5) Answer: 5%

Method: Reduction is 2 inches from 40. So the percentage reduction is $\frac{2}{40}$ ×100 = $\frac{1}{20}$ ×100 = 5%

(6) Answer: 300ml

Method: Since 50ml has 150mg. To find the number of ml required for 900mg we work out $\frac{900}{150}$ ×50 =6×50 = 300ml

(7) Answer: 230ml

Method: In one hour 40ml is infused. So in 5hours 45mins, 5.75×40 = 200 + 0.75×40 = 200 + 30 = 239ml (Note 5hrs 45mins = $5\frac{3}{4}$ hrs =5.75hrs)

(8) Answer: 3.45mg

Method: 1 mg = 1000mcg, so 3450mcg = 3450÷1000 =3.45mg

(9) Answer: (a) 145mg **(b)** 72.5mg

Method: (a) Her daily dose is 2.5×58 = 58×2 + 0.5×58 =116 +29 =145mg. **(b)** Her single dose is 145÷2 =72.5mg

(10) **Answer:** 50 drops/min

Method: drops/min $=\dfrac{600\ (ml)}{5}\times\dfrac{25}{60}=\dfrac{120\ (ml)}{1}\times\dfrac{25}{60}=\dfrac{2\ (ml)}{1}\times\dfrac{25}{1}=50$

(11) **Answer:** 90 tablets

Method: 3mg /day means 3 (1mg) tablets per day. This is equal to 3×30 =90 tablets.

(12) **Answer:** 1750

Method: 0.45litres = 450ml. This means the infusion lasts 450÷150 = 3 hours. Since the infusion starts at 1450 it will end 3 hours later that is at 1750.

(13) **Answer:** 60 drops/min

Method: drops/min $=\dfrac{300\ (ml)}{2.5}\times\dfrac{30}{60}=\dfrac{300\ (ml)}{2.5}\times\dfrac{1}{2}=\dfrac{120\ (ml)}{1}\times\dfrac{1}{2}=60$

(14) **Answer:** Yes
Method: Ratio of Total Cholesterol to HDL is **6:1.5** which simplifies **to 4: 1**, hence ratio as a fraction $=\dfrac{4}{1}=4$. **Yes, the patient meets the criteria**.

(15) **Answer:** 2ml

Method: Total volume of the solution including amount displaced = 5.5 + 0.5 = 6ml. Since 6ml now consists of 600mg this means the volume required to administer 200mg is: $\dfrac{200}{600}\times 6=\dfrac{2}{6}\times 6=2\times 1=2ml$

(16) **Answer:** 75 drops/min

Method: drops/min $=\dfrac{1200\ (ml)}{8}\times\dfrac{30}{60}=\dfrac{600\ (ml)}{4}\times\dfrac{1}{2}=\dfrac{150\ (ml)}{1}\times\dfrac{1}{2}=75$

(17) **Answer:** 750000mcg

Method: 0.75g = 0.75×1000 mg = 750mg. 750mg = 750×1000 =750000mcg

(18) Answer: 60%

Method: Increase in dose is 30mg. So increase in percentage from initial 50mg is $\frac{30}{50} \times 100 = 60\%$

(19) Answer: 50%

Method: Dose increase is 25mg. So percentage increase is $\frac{25}{50} \times 100 = \frac{1}{2} \times 100 = 50\%$

(20) Answer: 7.2mg

Method: Single dose = 20mcg×90 =1800mcg =1.8mg. Since the patient takes it qds then the total dose per day = 4×1.8 = 7.2mg

Some Useful Definitions and Reminders

Natural Numbers: are {1, 2, 3, 4, ...}

Whole Numbers: are {0, 1, 2, 3, ...}

Integers: These are whole numbers that include both positive and negative numbers including 0. So for example ....-5,-4,-3,-2, 0, 1, 2, 3, 4, ... are all integers.

Multiples: These are simply numbers in the multiplication tables.

For example the multiples of 6 are 6, 12, 18, 24, 30, ...

Factors: A factor is a number that divides exactly into another number as for example, the number 2 in the case of even numbers.

3 is a factor of 9, as 3 goes exactly into 9. Other factors of 9 are 1 and 9.

15, has two factors other than 15 and 1. The two factors are 5 and 3, since both these numbers go exactly into 15. **Example:** Find all the factors of 21. The factors are: 1, 3, 7 and 21 (since all these numbers divide exactly into 21)

Prime numbers: A prime number is a natural number that can be divided only by itself and by 1 (without a remainder). For example, 11 can be divided only by 1 and by 11. Prime numbers are whole numbers greater than 1. So for example the first 10 prime numbers are: 2, 3, 5, 7, 11, 13, 17, 19, 23 and 29. **Be careful that an odd number is not necessarily a prime number.** For example **9 is not a prime number** as its factors are 1, 3 and 9 and **prime numbers should have only two factors, 1 and the number itself. Also, note that 2 is a prime number, the only even number that can be divided by 1 and itself!**

Prime Factors: Some numbers can be written as a product of prime factors.

Example1: Write 28 as a product of prime factors.

Dividing 28 by the first prime factor 2 we are left with 14. Dividing 14 again by the first prime factor 2, we get 7. Now we can no longer divide 7 by the first prime factor 2. The next possible prime factor for 7 is obviously 7. **Hence 28 can be written as 2×2×7 or $2^2 \times 7$**

Example 2: Write the number 300 as a product of prime factors.

Step1: Divide by 300 by 2 to get 150,

Step 2: Divide 150 by 2 to get 75

Step 3: Divide 75 by 3 to get 25, Step 4: Divide 25 by 5 to get 5

Step 4: Divide 5 by 5 to get 1. Hence, **300 = 2×2×3×5×5 or $2^2 \times 3 \times 5^2$**

Another method of finding prime factors: Break down the required number at the top by dividing by prime factors starting with the lowest prime factor as shown below:

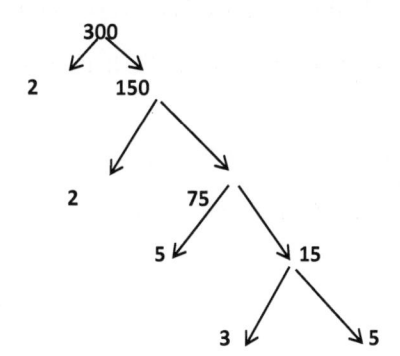

```
            300
           /   \
        2      150
              /   \
           2       75
          /       /  \
         5       15
                /  \
               3    5
```

Hence the product of prime factors for **300 = 2×2×3×5×5 or $2^2 \times 3 \times 5^2$**

Lowest Common Multiple (LCM)
This is essentially the smallest number that will divide exactly by the numbers given. Consider the examples below:

Example 1: Find the LCM of 15 and 45

One method is to find the multiples of both numbers and identify the lowest common multiple as shown below:

Multiples of 15 = 15, 30, **45**, 60, 90, ……..

Multiples of 45 = **45**, 90, 135, 180, ……

Clearly **45** (the highlighted number above) is the smallest number that is divisible by 15 and 45.

Example 2: Find the LCM of 10 & 15

First find the multiples of each number:

Multiples of 10 = 10, 20, **30**, 40, 50, 60, 70,…..

Multiples of 15 = 15, **30,** 45, 60, …..

You can see that **30** is the lowest common multiple since it is divisible both by 10 & 15.

Highest Common Factor (HCF)

This is the biggest number that will divide exactly into all the numbers given

Example 1: Find the HCF of 15 & 45

Method: Find the factors of each number given and then identify the biggest number that will divide into both these numbers as shown below:

Factors of 15 ={1, 3, 5, **15**}, Factors of 45 ={1, 3, 5, 9, **15**, 45}

You can see that **15** is the **highest common factor** which divides into **both** 15 and 45 exactly.

Example 2: Find the HCF of 8 and 32.

First find the factors of each number given

Factors of 8 ={1, 2, 4, **8**}, Factors of 32 = {1, 2, 4, **8**, 16, 32}

You can see that the number 8 is the highest **common** factor which divides into 8 and 32 exactly.

Square numbers and square roots

Squaring a number is simply multiplying a number by itself.

So 4^2 means 4 × 4 =16, 12^2 means 12 × 12 =144 and so on.

The square root is written like this $\sqrt{}$ and means finding a number which when multiplied by itself gives you the number inside the square root.

Example1: Find $\sqrt{16}$. The answer is clearly 4. Since 4×4 =16

Let us consider some other square roots.

$\sqrt{49}$ = 7, $\sqrt{121}$ =11, $\sqrt{100}$ =10, $\sqrt{225}$ = 15,

$\sqrt{256}$ = 16, $\sqrt{324}$ =18

Multiplying positive and negative numbers.

(+) × (+) = + (a plus number times a plus number gives us a plus number)

(+) × (−) = −- (a plus number times a minus number gives us a minus number)

(−) × (+) = − (a minus number times a plus number gives us a minus number)

(−) × (−) = + (a minus number times a minus number gives us a plus number)

Dividing positive and negative numbers.

(+) ÷ (+) = + (a plus number divided by a plus number gives us a plus number)

(+) ÷ (−) = − (a plus number divided by a minus number gives us a minus number)

(−) ÷ (+) = − (a minus number divided by a plus number gives us a minus number)

(−) ÷ (−) = + (a minus number times a minus number gives us a plus number)

Summary: For both multiplication and division, like signs gives us a plus sign and unlike signs gives a minus sign

Also when adding and subtracting it is worth knowing that:

When you add two minus numbers you get a bigger minus number.

Example 1: −4 − 6 = −10

When you add a plus number and a minus number you get the sign corresponding to the bigger number as shown below:

Example 2: +6 − 9 = −3, whereas, −6+9 = 3

When you subtract a minus from a plus or minus number you need to note the results as shown below:

Example 3: 6 − (− 3) we get 6+3 = 9 (since −(−3) = +3)

Example 4: 7 − (+3) we get 7 − 3 = 4 (since −(+3) = −3)

In this case note that − (−) = +. Also, +(−) = − and − (+) = −.

Finally you need to know the rules concerning the operation of numbers and one more symbol:

By operations we mean working out powers of numbers, multiplication, division, addition and subtraction. These operations need to be performed in the right order. Failing to do this might give you wrong results.

The rule taught traditionally is that of **BIDMAS.**

The **BIDMAS** rule is as follows:

> **(1) Always work out the Bracket(s) first**
> **(2) Then work out the Indices of a number (squares, cubes, square roots and so on)**
> (3) Now **M**ultiply and **D**ivide
> (4) Finally do the **A**ddition and **S**ubtraction.

Example 1: Work out 2(4+6) – 4

Work out the bracket first then times by 2 to get 2 × 10 =20. Finally take away 4 to get 16

So 2(4+6) – 4 =16

Example 2: $3 \times 4^2 + 13(7 - 2)$

The first part is 3 × 16 (we square before multiplying)

The second part is 13 × 5 (we do the brackets and then multiply)

The first part is thus 48 and the second part 65. Adding these two parts together we have 113.

So, $3 \times 4^2 + 13(7 - 2) = 113$

Printed in Great Britain
by Amazon.co.uk, Ltd.,
Marston Gate.